SURGERY - PROCEDURES, COMPLICATIONS, AND RESULTS

THE FUNDAMENTALS OF BARIATRIC SURGERY

SURGERY - PROCEDURES, COMPLICATIONS, AND RESULTS

Additional books in this series can be found on Nova's website under the Series tab.

Additional E-books in this series can be found on Nova's website under the e-book tab.

PUBLIC HEALTH IN THE 21ST CENTURY

Additional books in this series can be found on Nova's website under the Series tab.

Additional E-books in this series can be found on Nova's website under the e-book tab.

SURGERY - PROCEDURES, COMPLICATIONS, AND RESULTS

THE FUNDAMENTALS OF BARIATRIC SURGERY

SHAHZEER KARMALI
AND
DANIEL W. BIRCH
EDITORS

NOVA BIOMEDICAL
New York

For permission to use material from this book please contact us:
Telephone 631-231-7269; Fax 631-231-8175
Web Site: http://www.novapublishers.com

Library of Congress Cataloging-in-Publication Data

ISBN: 978-1-62417-732-3

Library of Congress Control Number: 2012955766

Published by Nova Science Publishers, Inc. † New York

To my wife, Saira for her incredible support and encouragement and to our two beautiful children Kiara and Noah, who are the joys of my life.

SK

To my wife Joanna and children William, Abby, Kate and Jack, all of whom I am fortunate to be with.

DWB

Contents

Preface

The prevalence of obesity, defined as a body mass index (BMI) > 30 kg/m2, has been steadily increasing in the United States and worldwide. Increased body mass is associated with an increased incidence of a wide range of medical problems affecting virtually every organ system. Each five-point increase in BMI over 25 kg/m2 is associated with a 30% increase in mortality. Furthermore, obesity also significantly affects quality of life, social functioning, and monetary health

The management of obesity is complex, often requiring an amalgamation of medical, dietary and psychological regimens to successfully tackle this multidimensional disease. Respectively, bariatric surgery has been utilized as a modality to manage morbid obesity and meta-analyses have demonstrated the efficacy of bariatric surgery in treating severe obesity and its associated co-morbidities An effect of this high utility benefit, is reflected in an exponential increase in the the number of bariatric operations performed in the United States (an 804 percent increase from 1998 to 2004. Hence, there are thousands of individuals yearly who have undergone or are undergoing bariatric surgery to manage morbid obesity.

Thus, it is critical for all general surgeons, whether they practice bariatric surgery or not to have a baseline understanding of the fundamentals underlying bariatric surgery pertaining to the preoperative assessment of the bariatric patient, the specifics of the commonly performed bariatric operations and an appreciation and understanding for managing potentially life threatening post operative complications. Herein, This textbook, *The Fundamentals of Bariatric Surgery*, is intended to provide the reader with a comprehensive overview of the management of the bariatric surgical patient. All of the contributors have been carefully selected as they each represent key opinion leaders in their own specific discipline regarding the assessment of the Bariatric patient and we hope that all the readers will get as much enjoyment in reading their contributions as we have had in preparing this seminal work.

Section 1: Introduction

In: The Fundamentals of Bariatric Surgery
Editors: Shahzeer Karmali and Daniel W. Birch
ISBN: 978-1-62417-732-3

Chapter 1

Bariatric Surgery: A Brief History in Time

C. J. de Gara
Professor of Surgery, Department of Surgery
University of Alberta, Edmonton, AB, Canada

Overview

- Identify the pioneers of bariatric surgery
- List the history of the procedures
- Highlight modifications to the various surgeries
- Indicate how their success and failures lead to these modifications
- Introduce the topics of medical tourism and revisional bariatric surgery

Introduction

The pioneers of bariatric surgery presaged the coming obesity epidemic of today. It is almost 60 years since bariatric surgery was first described in an attempt to address the life threatening disease, such as, diabetes, cardio vascular disease, sleep apnea, heightened cancer incidence, all associate with obesity and all leading to premature death [1]. We are now approaching the devastating reality that half of all Americans and Canadians are either overweight or obese[1]. It is claimed this is the first generation in humanity whose life expectancy will be greater than their children's [2].

The aim of this chapter will be to highlight the major bariatric surgical procedures as they evolved. The final section in the chapter will briefly outline the growing field of Revisional Bariatric surgery, as well as the challenges that "medical tourism" for bariatric procedures has led to [3].

Bariatric procedures are broadly divided into those that are restrictive, malabsorptive or a combination of the two.

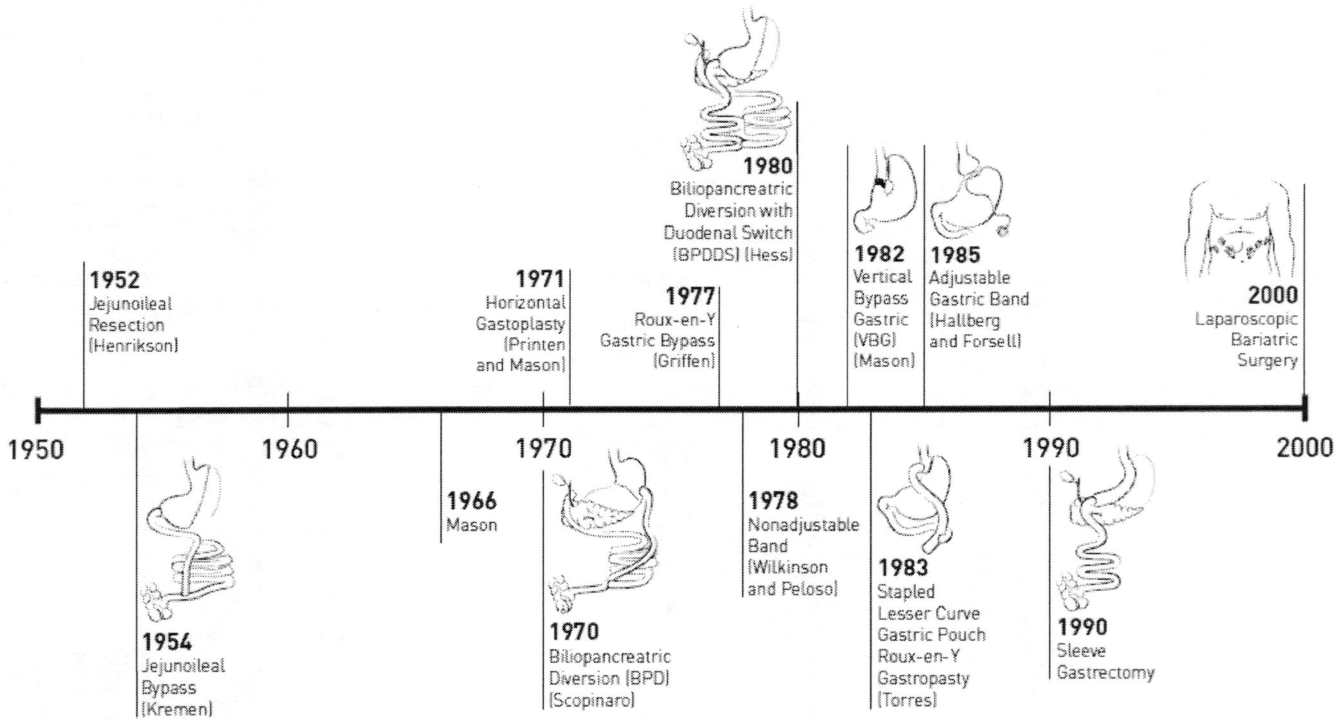

Figure 1. A timeline of bariatric surgical procedures.

The 50's Malabsorptive Procedures

In 1952, Dr Victor Henrikson [4] of Sweden carried out the first bariatric procedure. The operation involved the resection of 105 cm of small bowel in a single patient. In 1954, Dr Kremen et al. [5] from the University of Minnesota, carried out a series of experiments in dogs involving jejunoileal bypass (JIB) and subsequently carried out the procedure on a patient on April 9, 1954. Dr Payne and colleagues [6] modified the jejunoileal procedure to a jejunocolic anastomosis. However, this was associated with debilitating diarrhea, dehydration, and electrolyte imbalance (Figure 2).

Jejunoileal bypass remained popular in the 1960s and 70s but was associated with the blind loop syndrome, leading to bacterial overgrowth in the defunctioned limb which caused bloating and liver dysfunction occasionally leading to cirrhosis [7]. The procedure was associated with a significant protein malabsorption, vitamin deficiencies, and renal stones. Only about one third of patients had an acceptable post-operative outcome [8].

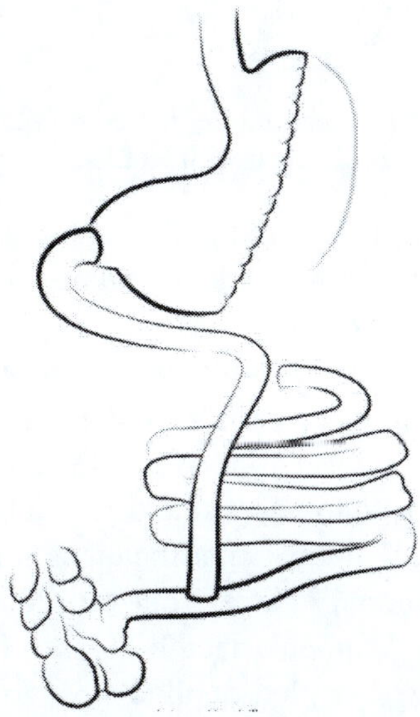

Figure 2. This diagram illustrates the procedure of a Jejunoileal Bypass first described in 1954. The operation involved dividing the small bowel and bypassing the majority of it with gastric and biliopancreatric juices entering the terminal ileum.

The 70's Biliopancreatic Diversion (BPD)

By combining malabsorptive and restrictive procedures, Dr Scopinaro and colleagues of Genoa, Italy developed biliopancreatic diversion in the mid 70s [9]. This procedure combined a subtotal gastrectomy with a Roux-en-Y procedure with a jejunoileal bypass. The procedure was sufficiently successful that Dr Scopinaro was able to report in 1998 on the long-term outcome in 2000 of 241 patients over 21 year period[9]. Weight loss was successful and maintained. In addition, the procedure had a dramatic effect on glycemic control in patients with Type II diabetes as well as controlling hypertension and hyperlipidemia.

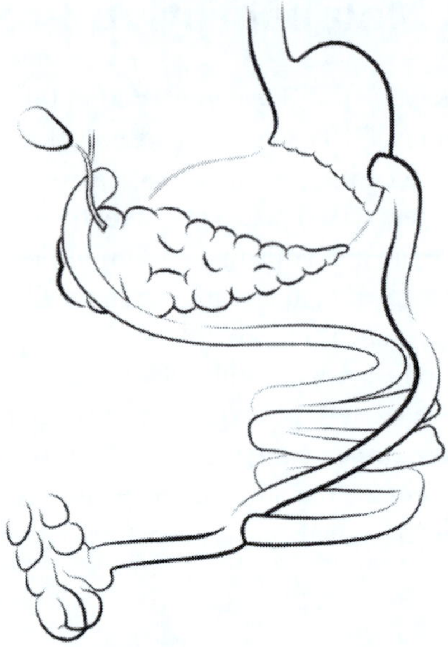

Figure 3. In the Biliopancreatic Diversion procedure, in addition to bypassing a considerable amount of small bowel, a hemi gastrectomy was preformed with Roux-en-Y type anastomosis.

Unfortunately, complications including diarrhea, foul-smelling stools, flatulence, anemia, stomal ulceration, protein malabsorption, and dumping syndrome were not uncommon, as well as significant vitamin D deficiencies.

In 1971, an attempt to avoid the morbidity associated with intestinal bypass developed a horizontal division of the upper stomach Printon and Mason [10], created a small pouch with a narrow channel along the greater curve to the rest of the stomach. Unfortunately, staple line dehiscence and pouch dilatation lead to unsatisfactory weight loss and weight regain.

Over the next several years, a number modifications including use of a mesh collar [11] ultimately lead to the most commonly carried out procedure of the day called the Vertical Banded Gastroplasty (Figure 3). As popularized by Mason [12], a narrow pouch of the upper stomach was created using a linear stapler, applied close to a Ewald tube. At the most distal end of the staple line, a circular stapler was used to create a window between the anterior and posterior aspects of the stomach around which a band of prolene mesh was encircle. The short term results of this procedure were very favorable with a gratifying weight reduction. However, at 5 years post operatively, failures were considerable with less than half the patients maintaining a satisfactory weight reduction [13]. These failures were mainly due to the dehiscence of the vertical staple line, thus returning the stomach to its normal size. Additionally, gastric pouch dilatation, band erosions and stricturing were also seen as complications of the procedure, but less commonly. In 1978, Wilkinson and Peloso of New Mexico [14] were the first to use a nonadjustable gastric band of Marlex mesh in the upper portion of the stomach.

Unfortunately, slippage of the band was common, leading to prolapse of the stomach both above and below the mesh. Additionally, erosion and stricturing causing esophageal and vomiting dilatation was noted. Eventual gastric pouch dilatation and weight regain would occur.

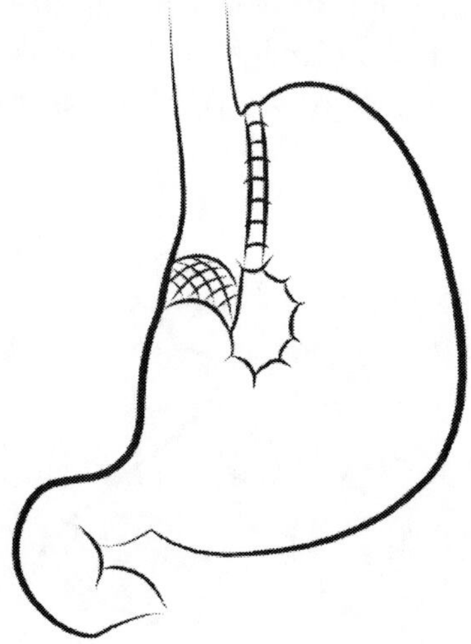

Figure 4. Shows the Vertical Band Gastroplasty. In this operation a right angle non cutting stapler was fired from the level of the ge-junction vertically for a length of approximately 10-12 cm, this separated the fundus of the stomach from the pouch and lesser curve of the stomach. At the distal of this staple firing a circular stapling device was used to develop a hole in the anterior and posterior walls of the stomach allowing a collar of mesh to be placed through this hole and encircle the lesser curve. This then created a small gastric pouch partially excluded from the rest of the stomach.

It was Hallberg and Forsell [15] of Sweden who in 1985 ushered in the concept of an inflatable gastric band. A procedure which remains popular to this day (Figure 6).

The 80's Biliopancreatic Diversion with Duodenal Switch (BPD/DS)

During the late 80s Hess and Marceau [16] developed a modification of the biliopancreatic diversion procedure by preserving the pylorus. The gastric resection was still carried out, but gastric emptying was maintained and the dumping syndrome eliminated. By preserving the duodenum, gastric acid was neutralized and ulcerations were reduced. The type of gastric resection was changed from the more traditional subtotal gastrectomy of the Billroth 2 type to a partial gastrectomy in which 70-80% of greater curve was resected; (the so called "sleeve" gastrectomy). In 1998, Hess and colleagues [17] published their experience on biliopancreatic diversion and duodenal switch procedure in 440 patients with 9-year of follow-up data. Similar weight loss was achieved, but far fewer marginal ulcerations and dumping syndrome, less liver and renal failure, and reduced electrolyte abnormalities were reported than with BPD alone. However, a number of revision procedures were necessary owing to excess weight loss.

The first gastric bypass was performed by Dr Edward E. Mason, in May 1966. The procedure involved dividing the proximal stomach horizontally, creating a small proximal gastric pouch, and a loop of jejunum was brought up to anastomose to this proximal pouch [18]. In 1977, Griffen, et al [19], introduced the Roux-en-Y configuration to replace the loop gastrojejunostomy. The major benefit was elimination of bile reflux into the gastric pouch.

This technique also added a malabsorptive component to the procedure. The original bypass operation was also associated with significant morbidity and mortality if anastomotic leakage occurred, which was somewhat reduced by carrying out a Roux-en-Y anastomosis.

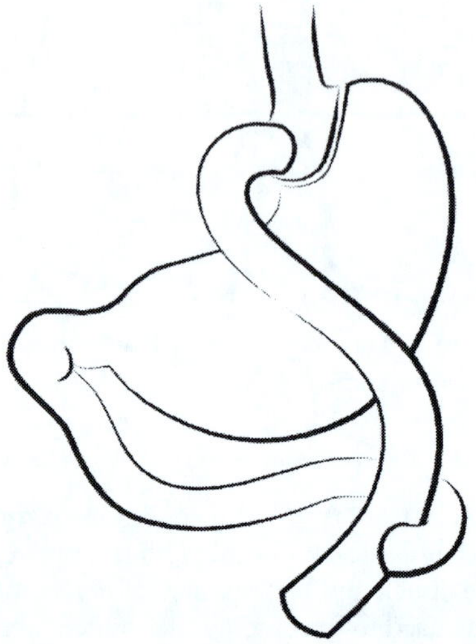

Figure 5. A Roux-en-Y Gastric Bypass in which a very small gastric pouch is created and a Roux-en-Y anastomosis with 100 cm of jejunum is brought up to the pouch and a 40 cm afferent biliopancreatic limb is anastomsed to the jejunum.

In 1983, Torres et al. [20] modified the gastric pouch based on the lesser curve of the stomach, with consequent better local blood supply and reduced chance of pouch dilatation. This modification has stood the test of time and is now the standard configuration (Figure 6).

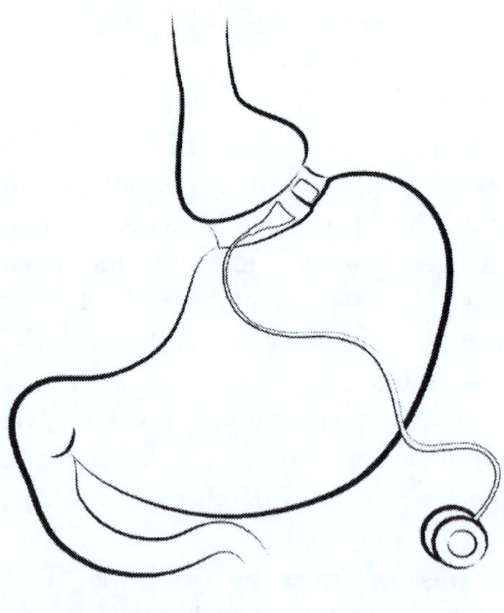

Figure 6. The Laparoscopic Adjustable Gastric Band involves encircling the most proximal portion of the stomach with a silastic collar that is inflatable through a subcutaneous port. The process of port inflation using anywhere between 5-10 cc of normal saline creates a significant restriction below a small gastric pouch.

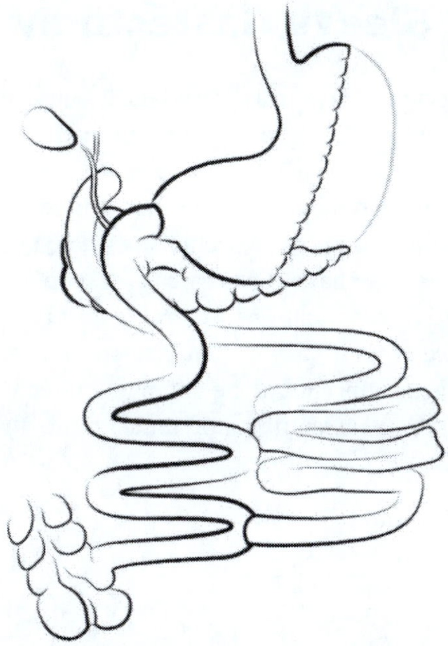

Figure 7. In the Biliopancreatic Diversion procedure, in addition to bypassing a considerable amount of small bowel, a hemi gastrectomy was preformed with Roux-en-Y type anastomosis.

Gastric Banding

Following a number of modifications, Forsell's band became known as the Swedish adjustable gastric band and was approved for use in Europe in 1996. Commercialization of various bands ensued including the Realize Band (Ethicon Endo Surgery Inc. Cincinnati, Ohio USA) and the LAP-BAND system (Allergen Inc, Irvin CA USA). These adjustable gastric bands have achieved considerable commercial success and there are many centres around the world now performing the procedure. It is essentially day surgery since these procedures can be done in under one hour laparoscopically with minimal perioperative morbidity. Unfortunately, adjustable gastric bands many not have the long-term success of other weight reduction strategies. While the procedure is quick to perform, close monitoring post-operatively is necessary with repeated band "fills" via subcutaneous port to achieve the necessary pouch reduction. There is risk of band slippage and band removal becomes necessary. Fortunately, once the band is removed, presuming no erosion, gastric function returns to normal. Because there are very few centres in North America where the cost of the band and its insertion are covered by the health system, these expenses have to be borne by the patient. Fees of $10,000 to $30,000 dollars are not unusual [21]. This has lead to a burgeoning "medical tourism" industry [3] where patients will travel to Mexico and South America for bariatric procedures. Significantly higher complications rates than might be expected in accredited and established bariatric surgical centres seem to occur. Additionally, the burden of band fills and post operative weight management falls to primary health care providers who may not have the necessary bariatric experience [3].

Sleeve Gastectomy

(Figure 8) Sleeve gastrectomy was originally described as a component of Biliopancreatric Diversion with Duodenal Switch procedure as originally described by Marceau and colleagues [21] in the 1990s. It became clear that this was an extremely effective operation, 80% gastric resection is carried out, and leaving a narrow gastrictube with antral and pyloric preservation was an extremely effective restrictive operation. While bleeding and staple line leakage have been areas of concern, advancements in stapler technology have reduced these complications to a relatively low incidence. Debate continues regarding the size of the sleeve with varying bougies from as small as 32-French up to 50-French, as well how much antrum should be retained. Given the relative novelty of this procedure, with measurable data extending not much more than 8 years, these questions remain to be fully answered.

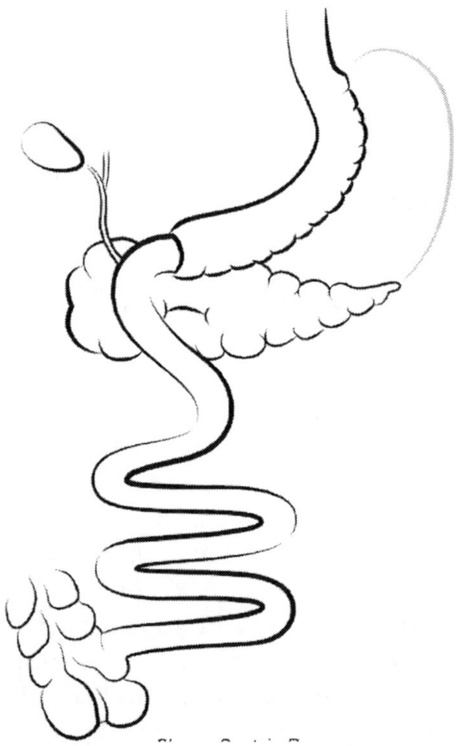

Figure 8. In the Sleeve Gastrectomy which was initially developed as a staged part of the biliopancreatic diversion with duodenal switch procedure, is now carried out as a single procedure laparoscopically in which over 80% of the greater curve is resected. A 32-French to 50-French orogastrically placed bougie is used to measure the remaining gastric sleeve.

The 90's and 2000's

A major revolution in bariatric surgery took place with the rapid adoption of Laparoscopic techniques in the 1990s. In 1992, the non adjustable gastric band was carried out laparoscopically followed by the adjustable gastric band in 1993, the vertical band gastroplasty, and laparoscopic Roux-en-Y gastroplasty. In 1999, Michelle Gagner [22] carried out the first duodenal switch operation laparoscopically and in 2003 laparoscopic sleeve gastrectomy was established. The impact of the laparoscope on the epidemic that represents obesity today has been considerable. It is now possible to carry out major upper gastrointestinal surgery with multiple staple lines and anastomosis and yet have patients be ready for discharge within 3 days of surgery. This would have been virtually unheard of at the time when a midline laparotomy was required in order to carry out these procedures.

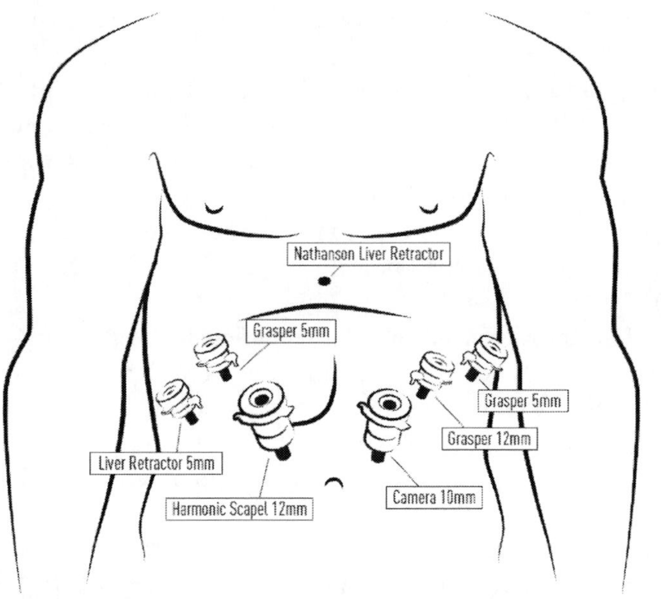

Figure 9. This diagram illustrate typical port placement in Laparoscopic Bariatric Surgery. A combination of 5–10–12–15 mm ports are used to allow instrumentation, camera and specimen removal. In the epigastrium a Nathanson retractor is placed via a stab incision, this allows for the left lateral segment of the liver to be retracted out of the field.

Critical to the establishment of bariatric surgery as a successful treatment of obesity has been the recognition of the importance of team based care. These procedures target a litany of comorbilities including such as Type II diabetes, hypertension, stroke, dyslipidemia, sleep apnea, joint disease and cancer. Articulated by Dr Arya Sharma [22] an experience team of nurses, dietitians, psychologists and physicians has clearly become a cornerstone of this therapy.

Inevitably, there will be failures of bariatric surgery. As a consequence, there is an evolving field of Revisional Bariatric Surgery [23]. While weight regain is one of the commonest indications for revisional surgery, mechanical problems such as gastric outlet obstruction, dumping syndrome or malabsorption, and vitamin deficiencies are also indications for surgery. Unfortunately, given the frequency of extensive adhesion formation that previous upper gastrointestinal surgery tends to produce, many of these revision operations do need to be carried out in an open setting, making the morbidity significantly higher than procedures done laparoscopically.

In conclusion, the 60 year history of bariatric surgery has seen a series of innovations developed and evolved by dedicated surgeons rising to the challenge that represents the morbid obesity epidemic. These have been and will continue to be necessary, until such a time as the medical management of this complex condition becomes effective.

References

[1] Lau, D, Douketis, J, Morrison K, et al 2006 Canadian clinical practice guidelines on the management and preventing of obesity in adults and children [summary], *CMAS* April 2007; Vol 176 8S1-S13.

[2] Olshansky, SJ, Passaro, D, et al A potential Decline in Life Expectancy in the United State in the 21st *Century: N Engl J Med* 2005; 352: 1138-1145. March 2005.

[3] Birch, D, Lan, V, Karmali, S et al Medical tourism in bariatric surgery. *The American Journal of Surgery* (2010) 199, 604-608.

[4] Henrikson V. [Kan tunnfarmsresektion forsvara som terapi mot fettsot? Nordisk Medicin 1952;47:744] Can small bowel resection be defended for therapy for obesity? *Obes Surg* 1994; 4:54-5.

[5] Kremen A, Linner J, Nelson C. An experimental evaluation of the nutritional importance of proximal and distal small intestine. *Ann Surg* 1945;140:439-44.

[6] Payne J, DeWind L, Commons R. Metabolic observations in patients with jejunocolic shunts. *AM J Surg* 1963; 106:2743-89.

[7] Brown R, O'Leary J, Woodward E. Hepatic effects of jejunoileal bypass for morbided obsesity. *AM J Surg* 1974; 127:53-8.

[8] Griffen W Jr, Young VL, Stevenson CC. A prospective comparison of gastric and jejunoileal bypass procedures for morbid obesity. *Ann Surg* 1977; 186(4): 500-9.

[9] Scopinaro N, Gianetti E, Adami G, et al. Biliopancreatic diversion for obesity at eighteen years. *Surgery* 1996; 119:261-8.

[10] Printen KJ, Mason EE. Gastric surgery or relief of morbid obesity. *Arch Surg* 1973; 106: 428-31.

[11] Gomez CA. Gastroplasty in the surgical treatment of morbid obesity. *AM J Clin Nutr* 1980; 33: 406-15.

[12] Mason EE, Vertical banded gastroplasty for obesity. *ArchSurg* 1982; 117:701-6.

[13] Mason EE, Maher JW, Scott DH, et al. Ten years of vertical banded gastroplasty for severe obesity. *Probl Gen Surg* 1992; 9(2): 280-9.

[14] Wilkinson LH, Peloso PA. Gastric (reservoir) reduction for morbid obesity. *Arch Surg* 1981; 116:602-5.

[15] Hallberg D, Forsell O. Ballongband vid behandling av massiv oberwikt. Svinsk Kiriurgi 1985; 344:106-8 [in Sweden].

[16] Lagace M, Marceau P, Marceau S, et al. Biliopancreatic diversion with a new type of gastrectomy: some previous conclusions revisited. *Obes Surg* 195; 5:411-8.

[17] Hess DS, Hess DW. Biolpancreatic diversion with a duodenal switch. *Obes Surg* 1998; 8:267-82.

[18] Mason EE, Ito C. Gastric bypass in obesity. *Surg Clin North AM* 167; 47(6):1345-51.

[19] Griffen W Jr, Younjg VL, Stevenson CC. A prospective comparison of gastric and jejunoileal bypass procedures for morbid obesity. *Ann Surg* 1977; 186(4): 500-9.
[20] Torres JC, Oca CF, Garrison RN, Roux-en-Y gastrojejunostomy from thelesser curvature, *South Med J* 1983; 76:1217-21
[21] Alden JF. Gastric and jejunoileal bypass. A comparison in the treatment of morbid obesity. *Arch Rug* 1977; 112(7):799-806.
[22] Hailoran K, Raj SP, Johnson-Stoklossa C, Sharma A, Birch D Income Status and Approval for Bariatric Surgery in Publicly Funded Regional Obesity Program; *Obesity Surgery*, Volume 21; 3, 373-378.
[23] Kellogg TA, Revision bariatric surgery, *Surg Clin North Am*, 2011 Dec; 91(6):1353-71.

In: The Fundamentals of Bariatric Surgery
Editors: Shahzeer Karmali and Daniel W. Birch
ISBN: 978-1-62417-732-3

Chapter 2

The Medical Complications of Obesity

Christian F. Rueda-Clausen and Raj Padwal
Department of Medicine, University of Alberta, Edmonton, AB, Canada

Abstract

Obesity is a complex chronic condition that substantially increases morbidity, mortality, medical costs and reduces quality of life. Obese patients often require comprehensive assessment and care, ideally delivered by a multidisciplinary team capable of prioritizing, integrating and managing the complex mixture of etiologies, comorbidities and complications unique to each obese patient. This chapter presents an overview of the etiology, pathophysiology and consequences of major obesity-related medical comorbidities commonly found in potential candidates for bariatric surgery.

Introduction

Numerous prospective observational studies have reported independent associations between overweight (BMI 25-29.9 kg/m^2) or obesity (BMI $\geq$ 30 kg/m^2) and increased mortality (Figure 1) [1, 2]. More specific markers of abdominal adiposity, such as abdominal circumference, have also shown to be associated with increased mortality, even after adjusting for BMI [3]. In addition, obesity independently increases the risk of developing numerous comorbidities (Figure 2) [4, 5]. In most cases, the strength of the association between body weight and the development of chronic pathologies is proportional to the degree of increased adiposity [6-8]. No randomized controlled trials have examined the effect of intentional weight loss on mortality risk. The best available evidence examining the relationship between intentional weight loss and mortality is from the Swedish Obesity Study [9]. In this high quality study, a matched observational design was used to compare 2010 patients who underwent bariatric surgery with 2037 controls. After 10 years of follow up, the surgery group had lost an average of 16% of initial body weight compared to a 2% weight gain in controls. Mortality rates in surgical patients were 71% (95% CI 54% to 92%) lower compared to controls. In addition to these data, numerous studies have demonstrated that intentional weight reductions in the order of 5-10% of initial body weight are consistently associated with improvements in obesity related comorbidities and quality of life [10-12].

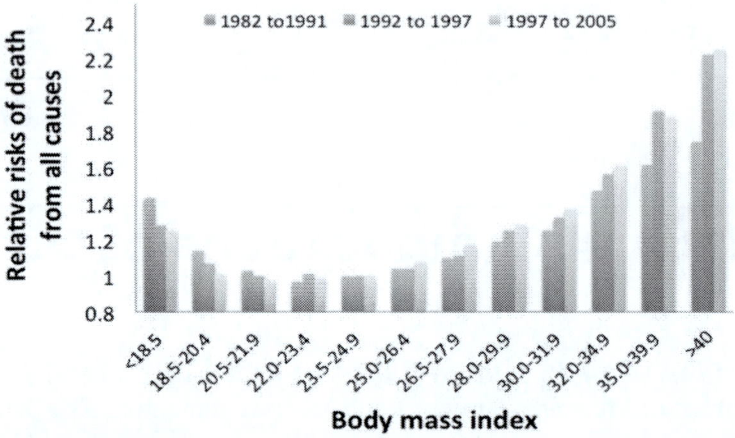

Data extracted from Calle *et al* [2]. This study included 317,875 healthy men and women. 69,229 subjects died during the 20-year follow-up period. Legend indicates year range of cohort entry. Participants included in this study had no baseline history of cancer (except non-melanoma skin cancer), heart disease, stroke, or respiratory disease (chronic bronchitis, emphysema, or asthma). They also had no current illness (of any type) and no history of weight loss (at least 10 lb) in the previous year. Relative risks were adjusted for age, sex, level of education, physical activity, alcohol use, marital status, aspirin use, fat consumption, vegetable consumption, race, and use of estrogen-replacement therapy (in women). Subjects with a BMI of 23.5 to 24.9 kg/m^2 were used as reference category.

Figure 1. Relative risks of death from all causes according to body-mass index.

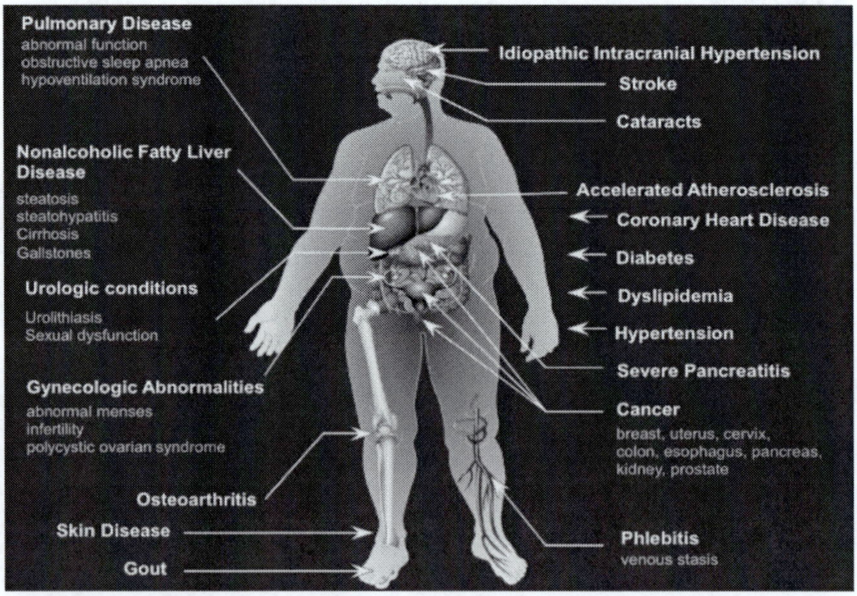

Adapted from, Canadian Obesity Network training material (www.obesitynetwork.com)

Figure 2. Common medical complications associated with obesity.

Cardiovascular Complications of Obesity

Obesity is associated with a number of cardiovascular complications including hypertension, coronary artery disease, cerebrovascular disease, heart failure, endothelial dysfunction, venous insufficiency and atrial fibrillation.

Hypertension

As adiposity increases, so does the risk of high blood pressure and these two risk factors commonly coexist in patients with the metabolic syndrome (see below). The risk of hypertension in the population that is attributable to excess body weight is estimated to be 25-30% [13].

The pathogenesis of hypertension in obese individuals is complex and poorly understood. Activation of the renin-angiotensin system, increased leptin levels, higher sympathetic nervous system activity, enhanced renal sodium retention and sleep apnea are all thought to contribute. Lifestyle modification to induce weight loss is an effective treatment for hypertension in obese individuals. A meta-analysis of 25 RCTs reported that a 5.1 kg weight loss leads to a 4.4 mmHg reduction in systolic blood pressure and a 3.6 mmHg reduction in diastolic blood pressure [14].

Endothelial Dysfunction and Atherosclerosis

One of the major putative pathophysiological mechanisms linking obesity with atherosclerosis is endothelial dysfunction [15]. The inappropriate secretion of pro-inflammatory factors (also known as adipokines) from the adipocyte (such as interleukin 6, tumor necrosis factor alpha, adiponectin and hepatocyte growth factor) leads to insulin resistance, inflammation and vascular wall remodeling [16, 17]. This results in an imbalance between oxidative stress and antioxidant mechanisms and, ultimately, impaired vascular homeostasis and endothelial dysfunction. In addition, conditions commonly associated with obesity such as hyperinsulinemia and vascular smooth muscle proliferation further contribute to vascular dysfunction.

Coronary Heart Disease

Obesity, particularly visceral adiposity, independently increases the risk of acute coronary events. Both increased BMI and increased visceral adiposity are independent risk factors for coronary disease. In the INTERHEART study, a case-control study of 27 098 subjects in 52 countries, the top quintile of BMI was associated with an increased risk of myocardial infarction (OR 1.4; 95% CI 1.3-1.6) compared to the bottom quintile, but this association became non-significant after adjustment for waist circumference and other independent cardiovascular risk factors (Figure 3) [18, 19].

In contrast, a higher degree of central adiposity (either waist-to-hip ratio or waist circumference) was independently associated with the risk of myocardial infarction even after adjustment for BMI (Figure 3). These data demonstrate, that, although BMI is an important risk factor for coronary heart disease, indexes of central adiposity more accurately predict the risk of this important complication.

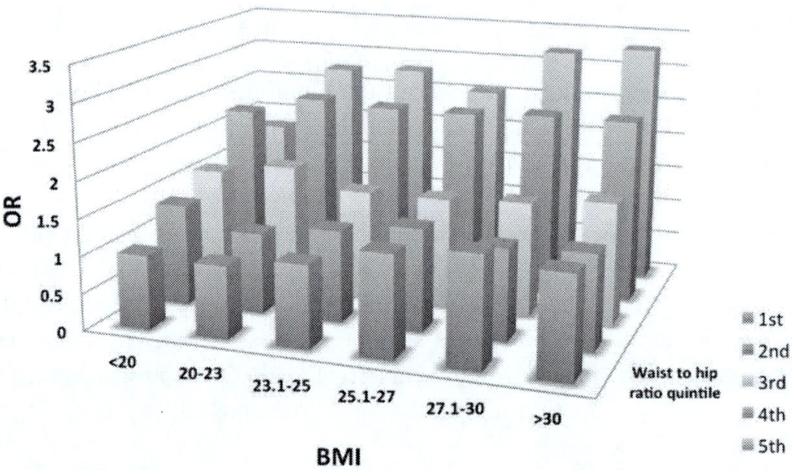

Independent of BMI, the presence of an increased waist-to-hip ratio is associated with a greater risk of having a myocardial infarction. Subjects in the first waist to hip quintile and a body-mass index <20 were used as reference category. Adapted from Yusuf *et al* [19].

Figure 3. Independent association between waist-to-hip ratio and risk of myocardial infarction by BMI level.

Cerebrovascular Disease

Obesity is a well-recognized risk factor for ischemic stroke. [20-24], [25]. A recent meta-analysis that included data from over 2 million participants [26] reported that the risk of ischemic stroke was increased in both overweight RR 1.22 (95%CI 1.05–1.41) and obese RR 1.64 (95%CI 1.36–1.99).

In addition a large study that include data from 4 cohorts involving 76,227 Chinese adults showed that each increase of 2 kg/m^2 in BMI caused a 18.8% increase in RR of ischemic stroke [27].

Pulmonary/Respiratory Complications of Obesity

A variety of respiratory changes are associated with obesity, ranging from small reductions in ventilation, with no effect on gas exchange, to more serious conditions, such as hypercapnic respiratory failure (Figure 4). Recent studies have also linked obesity (which itself is a low grade inflammatory state) and other chronic inflammatory respiratory conditions, such as asthma.

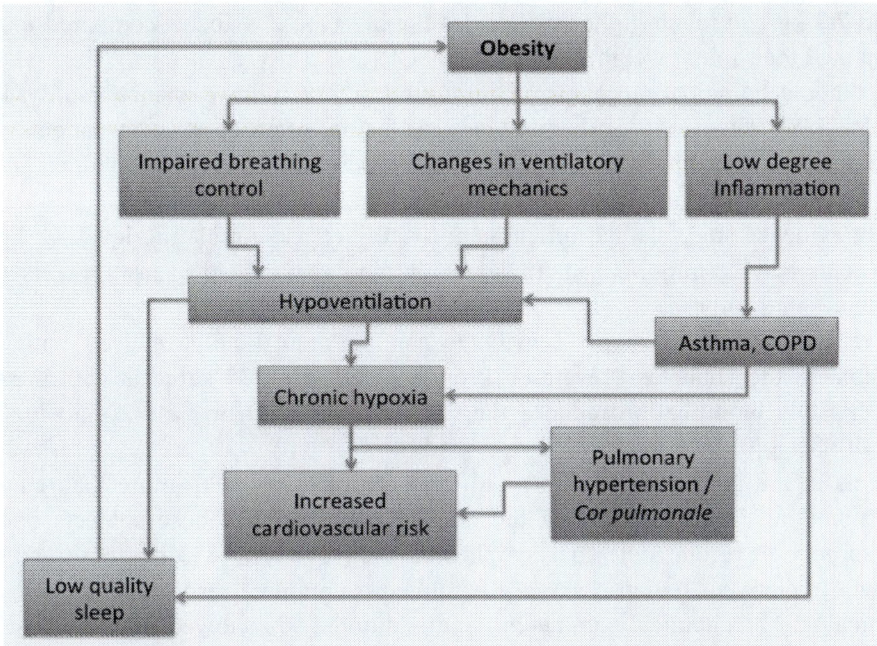

Figure 4. Main proposed mechanism linking obesity and pulmonary pathology.

Two of the most serious complications resulting from obesity are sleep apnea and obesity hypoventilation syndrome. The obesity hypoventilation syndrome is defined as the combination of obesity (defined as a body mass index >30 kg/m^2) and awake arterial hypercapnia ($PaCO_2$ >45 mmHg) in the absence of other known causes of hypoventilation [28]. This condition was initially described as "Pickwickian syndrome", named after a character in the Charles Dickens novel, "The Posthumous Papers of the Pickwick Club". Common clinical manifestations of sleep apnea include excessive daytime sleepiness, fatigue, and morning headaches. Hypoxemia-induced erythrocytosis, pulmonary hypertension and *cor pulmonale* are common sequelae. Patients who also are afflicted with the obesity hypoventilation syndrome exhibit daytime hypercapnia, hypoventilation, and hypoxemia during wakefulness. Although both conditions are independently associated with an increased risk of death, obesity hypoventilation syndrome can be particularly deadly. In 277 hospitalized severely obese patients, those with obesity hypoventilation syndrome had a 4.0-fold (95% CI 1.5 to 10.4) higher risk of mortality at 23 months compared to subjects who did not have this condition [29].

Type 2 Diabetes

The association between obesity, insulin resistance and type 2 diabetes mellitus has been extensively described over the past decades [30-36]. More than 80% of the risk associated with type 2 diabetes can be attributed to excess adiposity (especially centrally deposited adipose tissue) and the risk of type 2 diabetes increases substantially as weight increases. For example, in an analysis of 114 281 women enrolled in the Nurses Health Study, subjects that gained 5.0-7.9 kg had much higher risk of developing type 2 diabetes compared to subjects that maintained their initial weight (RR 1.9; 95% CI 1.5-2.3) [37].

The pathophysiological mechanisms linking obesity, insulin resistance and dysglycemia are complex [38]. These two cardiovascular risk factors often co-exist in patients with the metabolic syndrome along with hypertension and dyslipidemia. Such individuals also often exhibit low grade inflammation and a prothrombotic state.

Recent evidence suggests that inflammation and increase circulating levels of lipids and free fatty acids may be important intermediates in the development of insulin resistance and type 2 diabetes in the obese [39].

The risk of developing type 2 diabetes can be dramatically reduced with lifestyle modification. In the Diabetes Prevention Program RCT of 3234 subjects with prediabetes, intensive lifestyle modification reduced the risk of progression to type 2 diabetes by 58% (95% CI 48-68%)[40].

Subjects in the intensive lifestyle modification arm lost 4.1 kg more than controls. In addition, numerous studies following the clinical evolution of obese subjects undergoing bariatric surgery A recent meta-analysis showed that, overall, 78% of obese and diabetic patients who underwent bariatric surgery exhibited a complete resolution of their diabetes (both clinical and biochemical parameters) and additional 9% showed improvement of their glucose homeostasis parameters including fasting glucose, HbA1c and insulin levels [41].

Urologic Complications of Obesity

A growing body of evidence has demonstrated that overweight and obesity are major contributing factors to many common urological conditions including urolithiasis, chronic kidney disease, benign prostatic hyperplasia, urinary incontinence, sexual dysfunction (both in male and female) and androgen deficiency syndrome.

Moreover, the presence of obesity has also been associated to an increased incidence and poor prognosis of such urological conditions as Fournier's gangrene and complex urinary tract infections [42-44].

Several pathophysiological changes associated with obesity such as insulin resistance, hyperinsulinemia, increased renal ammonium production, decreased urinary pH and hypocitraturia all may contribute towards the development of calcium oxalate stones in these patients.

Moreover, a larger body size may also result in increased urinary excretion of uric acid and oxalate, which predisposes towards the development of calcium oxalate kidney stones [42] (Table 1).

Overweight and obesity not only increase the prevalence of chronic urologic conditions but also restrict the number of therapeutic alternative available for a patient with a define urological complication. Obese women with neurogenic bladder or urinary incontinence, for instance, are sub-optimally treated with urethral or suprapubic catheters because morbid obesity prevents self-catheterization (due to mechanical issues) or surgical re-construction (due to the elevated surgical risk).

Table 1. Adjusted relative risk for symptomatic urolithiasis according to the presence of obesity or weight gain

	Men (40-75 Yrs)	**Younger Women (27-44 Yrs)**	**Older Women (34-59 Yrs)**
Body weight			
>100 Vs. <68.2 Kg	1.44 (1.11-1.86)	1.92 (1.59-2.31)	1.89 (1.52-2.36)
Weight gain during adulthood (vs. no weight gain)			
>15.9 Kg since 21 Yrs of age	1.39 (1.14-1.70)	--	--
>15.9 Kg since 18 Yrs of age	--	1.70 (1.40-2.05)	1.82 (1.50-2.21)
BMI			
>30 vs. 12-22.9	1.33 (1.08-1.63)	2.09 (1.77-2.48)	1.90 (1.61-2.25)
>35 vs. 21-23	--	2.28 (1.87-2.79)	2.27 (1.87-2.81)
Waist circumference			
>109.2cm vs. <86.4cm	1.48 (1.13-1.93)	--	--
>101.6cm vs. <78.7cm	--	1.94 (1.49-5.52)	1.71 (1.40-2.10)

Data presented as adjusted RR (95% CI), variables use for models included age, use of thiazide diuretics, alcohol use, calcium supplement use, and dietary intake of fluid, animal protein, calcium, magnesium, potassium, sodium, and vitamin C. Data extracted from Taylor *et al* 2005 [42].

Gastrointestinal Complications of Obesity

Several studies have illustrated a strong direct association between body mass index and gastroesophageal reflux disease (GERD). A meta-analysis of nine studies evaluating the association between BMI and GERD [45] concluded that, compared to subjects with normal BMI, the pooled adjusted odds ratios for GERD symptoms in subjects with overweight was 1.43 [95% CI 1.15 -1.77] and for subjects with obesity was 1.94 [95% CI 1.46-2.56] [45].

Other gastrointestinal conditions associated with obesity include nonalcoholic steatohepatitis (NASH), erosive esophagitis, cholelithiasis and constipation. NASH is a particularly important potential consequence of excess visceral adiposity, type 2 diabetes, dyslipidemia and the metabolic syndrome.

The pathogenesis is thought to result from increased circulating levels of free fatty acids released from dysfunctional and insulin-resistant adipocytes, which result in the accumulation of triglyceride-derived toxic metabolites in the liver. This leads to the subsequent migration of inflammatory cells and the activation of inflammatory pathways [46-48]. Chronic hepatitis is associated with an increased risk of cirrhosis, hepatocelullar carcinoma and emerging data indicate that weight loss induced by bariatric surgery may mitigate the presence and progression of NASH [49].

The risk of developing gallstones is also increased in subjects with obesity [50]. This probably due to a combination of biochemical and dynamic factors such as increased saturation of gallbladder bile with cholesterol and possible gallbladder stasis. Interestingly, despite the normalization in bile composition after losing weight, rapid and substantial weight loss is a risk factor for cholesterol crystal and gallstone formation[51, 52]. Obese subjects undergoing bariatric surgery have gallstone incidence rates that are 15- to 25-fold higher than in the general obese population during the first month after surgery, however, only one-third of the subjects will be symptomatic and only half of those who are symptomatic will require further surgical management [53].

Commonly proposed mechanisms underlying gallstone formation after bariatric surgery include transitory biliary cholesterol saturation secondary to increased cholesterol mobilization, bile stasis due to reduced caloric intake and increased stone nucleation due to changes in bile arachidonate and glycoprotein concentrations [53].

Osteomuscular Complications of Obesity

Chronic osteomuscular conditions (particularly chronic pain) are common in obese individuals. A cross-sectional study of 3637 Americans, reported that subjects with obesity exhibit an increased risk of chronic pain (odds ratio (OR)=1.8 for class I, 1.9 for class II and 2.3 for class III obesity) compared to normal-weight subjects [54]. Obese subjects are also more likely to have pain in multiple body parts.

Among Hispanic-American subjects with overweight and obesity and presenting with chronic pain, the number of painful areas and the severity of the pain were directly correlated to the severity of excess weight [55](Figure 5).

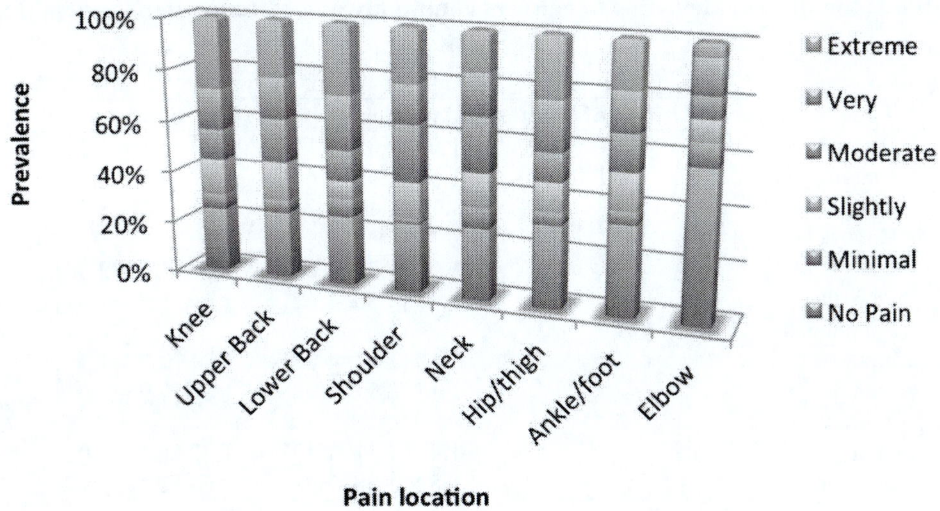

Data extracted from Zettel-Watson et al.[55].

Figure 5. Frequency and severity of chronic pain reported in obese subjects.

The pathophysiological mechanisms linking overweight and obesity and the presence of chronic osteomuscular pain are multiple and rather complex. Osteoarthritis is a chronic disease characterized by the gradual degradation, inflammation and remodeling of articular cartilage leading to a failure to support the mechanical demands of the joints. Large longitudinal studies have demonstrated that obesity increases the risk of osteoarthritis in the lower body [56, 57], which is due not only to increased biomechanical stress [58] but also to the increased presence of other osteomuscular comorbidities such sarcopenia and impaired cartilage homeostasis [59, 60].

Weight reductions post-bariatric surgery can alleviate joint pain - close to 40% of all obese subjects with joint pain reported were pain-free 10 months after undergoing surgery [61, 62].

Obesity and Neoplastic Syndromes

Excess adiposity is associated with an increased risk of cancer incidence, earlier relapse in treated subjects and diminished overall survival after diagnosis [63]. Compared to subjects with normal weight, severely obese men and women have a notably increased risk of death from all cancers combined (52% [95%CI 13-105%] increased risk for men and 62% [95%CI 40-87%] for women) [64].

In fact, it has been estimated that close to 20% (for women) and 14% (for men) of all cancer mortalities can be attributed to obesity [64]. Excess adiposity primarily increases the risk for breast, gastrointestinal, gynecological and genitourinary malignancies (Table 2).

Table 2. Incidence rate ratios of cancers commonly associated with overweight and obesity

Type of cancer	# of studies	Overweight	Obesity
Breast*	14	1.08 [1.03–1.14]	1.13 [1.05–1.22]
Endometrial*	10	1.53 [1.45–1.61]	3.22 [2.91–3.56]
Ovarian	9	1.18 [1.12–1.23]	1.28 [1.20–1.36]
Colorectal	12		
men		1.51 [1.37–1.67]	1.95 [1.59–2.39]
women		1.45 [1.30–1.62]	1.66 [1.52–1.81]
Esophageal	1		
men		1.13 [1.02–1.26]	1.21 [0.97–1.52]
women		1.15 [0.97–1.36]	1.20 [0.95–1.53]
Kidney	5		
men		1.40 [1.31–1.49]	1.82 [1.61–2.05]
women		1.82 [1.68–1.98]	2.64 [2.39–2.90]
Pancreatic	6		
men		1.28 [0.94– 1.75]	2.29 [1.65–3.19]
women		1.24 [0.98–1.56]	1.60 [1.17–2.20]

Data adapted from Guh *et al.*[83] and presented as incidence rate ratios (IRRs) [95%CI]. *Postmenopausal women only.

Breast Cancer

Breast cancer in postmenopausal women is among the most extensively studied neoplastic condition associated with overweight (IRR 1.08 95%co 1.03-1.14) and obesity (IRR 1.13 95%CI 1.05-1.22) [65]. A growing body of evidence also suggests that obesity is associated with poor prognosis in women diagnosed with early-stage breast cancer [66]. In addition, compared with normal weight women, women who are overweight or obese at the time of diagnosis have an increased risk or recurrence and have higher mortality rates [67, 68]. Although gaining some weight after being diagnosed with cancer is generally perceived as an indicator of good prognosis for many types of cancers, gaining weight after the diagnosis may be associated with poor prognosis in subjects with breast cancer [69].

Colorectal Cancer

A recent meta-analysis that included 31 studies and over 70.000 subjects concluded that compared to normal weight subjects, the risk of colorectal cancer is significantly increased in subjects with obesity, regardless of whether obesity was defined by BMI (OR 1.19 [95% CI 1.11-1.29]) or abdominal circumference (OR 1.45 [95% CI 1.31-1.61]) [70]. Moreover, there is evidence for a dose-response relationship between obesity and the risk of colorectal cancer: for every 2 kg/m^2 increase in BMI the risk of colorectal cancer increased by 7% (95% CI 4-10%) and for every 2-cm increase in waist circumference, the risk increased by 4% (95% CI 2-5%) [70].

Pancreatic Cancer

After adjusting for confounding factors, such as diabetes and pancreatitis, overweight and obese subjects have an increased risk of pancreatic cancer OR 1.67 [95%CI 1.20-2.34] and 2.58 [95% CI 1.70-3.90] respectively. Moreover, being overweight or obese at the time of the diagnosis is associated with decreased survival regardless of disease stage and tumor resection status (HR 1.26 [95% CI 0.94-1.69] for overweight and 1.86 [95% CI 1.35-2.56] for obesity) [71].

Dermatologic Complications of Obesity

Both the dermatological manifestations of obesity as well as common dermatological conditions that are aggravated by obesity are commonly overlooked despite the fact that these conditions can have important impact on the quality of life obese subjects [72, 73]. The types of dermatological manifestations/complications of obesity are diverse and can be categorized into mechanical, endocrine, infectious and inflammatory mechanisms [74-76] (Table 3).

Table 3. Common non-neoplastic skin disorders associated with or aggravated by obesity

	Common obesity manifestations or comorbidities	Conditions aggravated by obesity
Metabolic		
	Acanthosis nigricans	Tophaceous gout
	Acrochordons	
	Keratosis pilaris	
	Hyperandrogenism	
	Hirsutism	
Mechanical		
	Cellulite	Lymphedema
	Striae distensae	Chronic venous insufficiency/Ulcers
	Fat redistribution	Plantar hyperkeratosis
	Adiposis dolorosa	Adiposis dolorosa
		Poor healing of acute and chronic wounds
Infectious		
	Intertrigo	Erysipelas
	Candidal intertrigo	Necrotizing cellulitis/fasciitis
	Dermatophytes	
	Folliculitis	
	Skin tags	
	Furunculosis	
Inflammatory		
	Hidradenitis suppurativa	Psoriasis
		Acne

Psychological/Psychiatric and Social Complications of Obesity

The fact that obese patients have significantly poorer quality of life than their normal weight counterparts is not surprising considering the number of serious comorbidities associated with obesity. Interestingly, many obese subjects, and particularly those seeking for help, are more likely to attribute their impaired quality of life to psychological /emotional/social factors rather than to other comorbidities [77]. Not surprisingly, subjects with morbid obesity are commonly described as depressed, anxious, having poor impulse control and possessing low self-esteem [78]. Obese patients have a higher prevalence (40% to 50%) of psychiatric disorders than the normal weight population [79]. In addition the prevalence of eating disorders and certain psychological characteristics and personality traits (e.g. passive-aggressive) known to reduce the chance of successful weight management are extremely high in the obese population [80]. However, it is not clear whether the presence of these psychiatric conditions affects the outcomes of subjects pursuing weight management, or whether the normal history of the psychiatric disease is different in subjects with overweight and obesity [77]. Bariatric surgery candidates do have the tendency to deny psychological problems in order to be approved for surgery. Therefore, performing a comprehensive psychological assessment and developing an individualized psychosocial treatment plan in selected bariatric surgery candidates in whom mental health challenges exist is fundamental to the care of these patients [78, 81]. The negative social implications of obesity are closely related to the presence of psychological comorbidities. For example, obese individuals are more likely to be targets of stigmatization and discrimination throughout their lives, beginning in early childhood. These challenges are also commonly found in medical settings [82]. Physicians, nurses, dietitians, psychologists, medical students and even specialists in obesity management can commonly express negative attitudes toward overweight patients. Obese patients are more likely to avoid medical care and to delay important preventive health care services and cancel medical appointments to avoid experiencing weight bias from health care providers.

Conclusion

Obesity is a very complex, multifactorial and chronic condition that can lead to medical complications compromising almost every organ and system in the body. Overall, the prevalence and severity of most medical complications of obesity are directly associated with the severity of the obesity problem. Therefore, efforts aiming at sustained reductions in bodyweight may have substantial impact morbidity and mortality in the obese.

References

[1] Reis JP, Macera CA, Araneta MR, Lindsay SP, Marshall SJ, Wingard DL. Comparison of overall obesity and body fat distribution in predicting risk of mortality. *Obesity* (Silver Spring). 2009 Jun;17(6):1232-9.

[2] Calle EE, Teras LR, Thun MJ. Obesity and mortality. *N Engl J Med*. 2005 Nov 17;353(20):2197-9.

[3] Bigaard J, Tjonneland A, Thomsen BL, Overvad K, Heitmann BL, Sorensen TI. Waist circumference, BMI, smoking, and mortality in middle-aged men and women. *Obes Res*. 2003 Jul;11(7):895-903.

[4] Chen J. Multiple signal pathways in obesity-associated cancer. O*bes Rev*. 2011 Dec;12(12):1063-70.

[5] Hankey GJ. Nutrition and the risk of stroke. *Lancet* Neurol. 2012 Jan;11(1):66-81.

[6] Benraouane F, Litwin SE. Reductions in cardiovascular risk after bariatric surgery. *Curr Opin Cardiol*. 2011 Nov;26(6):555-61.

[7] Kenchaiah S, Gaziano JM, Vasan RS. Impact of obesity on the risk of heart failure and survival after the onset of heart failure. *Med Clin North Am*. 2004 Sep;88(5):1273-94.

[8] Ni Mhurchu C, Parag V, Nakamura M, Patel A, Rodgers A, Lam TH. Body mass index and risk of diabetes mellitus in the Asia-Pacific region. *Asia Pac J Clin Nutr*. 2006;15(2):127-33.

[9] Sjostrom L, Narbro K, Sjostrom CD, Karason K, Larsson B, Wedel H, et al. Effects of bariatric surgery on mortality in Swedish obese subjects. *N Engl J Med*. 2007 Aug 23;357(8):741-52.

[10] Kaukua J, Pekkarinen T, Sane T, Mustajoki P. Health-related quality of life in obese outpatients losing weight with very-low-energy diet and behaviour modification--a 2-y follow-up study. *Int J Obes Relat Metab Disord*. 2003 Oct;27(10):1233-41.

[11] Klingemann J, Pataky Z, Iliescu I, Golay A. Relationship between quality of life and weight loss 1 year after gastric bypass. *Dig Surg*. 2009;26(5):430-3.

[12] Kolotkin RL, Crosby RD, Williams GR, Hartley GG, Nicol S. The relationship between health-related quality of life and weight loss. *Obes Res*. 2001 Sep;9(9):564-71.

[13] Wilson PW, D'Agostino RB, Sullivan L, Parise H, Kannel WB. Overweight and obesity as determinants of cardiovascular risk: the Framingham experience. *Arch Intern Med*. 2002 Sep 9;162(16):1867-72.

[14] Neter JE, Stam BE, Kok FJ, Grobbee DE, Geleijnse JM. Influence of weight reduction on blood pressure: a meta-analysis of randomized controlled trials. *Hypertension*. 2003 Nov;42(5):878-84.

[15] Tesauro M, Cardillo C. Obesity, blood vessels and metabolic syndrome. *Acta Physiol* (Oxf). 2011 Sep;203(1):279-86.

[16] Lobo RA. The risk of stroke in postmenopausal women receiving hormonal therapy. *Climacteric*. 2009;12 Suppl 1:81-5.

[17] Towfighi A, Zheng L, Ovbiagele B. Weight of the obesity epidemic: rising stroke rates among middle-aged women in the United States. *Stroke*. 2010 Jul;41(7):1371-5.

[18] Yusuf S, Hawken S, Ounpuu S, Dans T, Avezum A, Lanas F, et al. Effect of potentially modifiable risk factors associated with myocardial infarction in 52 countries (the INTERHEART study): case-control study. *Lancet*. 2004 Sep 11-17;364(9438):937-52.

[19] Yusuf S, Hawken S, Ounpuu S, Bautista L, Franzosi MG, Commerford P, et al. Obesity and the risk of myocardial infarction in 27,000 participants from 52 countries: a case-control study. *Lancet*. 2005 Nov 5;366(9497):1640-9.

[20] Yatsuya H, Toyoshima H, Yamagishi K, Tamakoshi K, Taguri M, Harada A, et al. Body mass index and risk of stroke and myocardial infarction in a relatively lean population: meta-analysis of 16 Japanese cohorts using individual data. *Circ Cardiovasc Qual Outcomes*. 2010 Sep;3(5):498-505.

[21] Chen Z, Yang G, Offer A, Zhou M, Smith M, Peto R, et al. Body mass index and mortality in China: a 15-year prospective study of 220 000 men. *Int J Epidemiol*. 2012 Jan 31.

[22] Hu G, Tuomilehto J, Silventoinen K, Sarti C, Mannisto S, Jousilahti P. Body mass index, waist circumference, and waist-hip ratio on the risk of total and type-specific stroke. *Arch Intern Med*. 2007 Jul 9;167(13):1420-7.

[23] Suk SH, Sacco RL, Boden-Albala B, Cheun JF, Pittman JG, Elkind MS, et al. Abdominal obesity and risk of ischemic stroke: the Northern Manhattan Stroke Study. *Stroke*. 2003 Jul;34(7):1586-92.

[24] Yatsuya H, Folsom AR, Yamagishi K, North KE, Brancati FL, Stevens J. Race- and sex-specific associations of obesity measures with ischemic stroke incidence in the Atherosclerosis Risk in Communities (ARIC) study. *Stroke*. 2010 Mar;41(3):417-25.

[25] Goldstein LB, Bushnell CD, Adams RJ, Appel LJ, Braun LT, Chaturvedi S, et al. Guidelines for the primary prevention of stroke: a guideline for healthcare professionals from the American Heart Association/American Stroke Association. Stroke. 2011 Feb;42(2):517-84.

[26] Strazzullo P, D'Elia L, Cairella G, Garbagnati F, Cappuccio FP, Scalfi L. Excess body weight and incidence of stroke: meta-analysis of prospective studies with 2 million participants. *Stroke*. 2010 May;41(5):e418-26.

[27] Zhou BF. Effect of body mass index on all-cause mortality and incidence of cardiovascular diseases--report for meta-analysis of prospective studies open optimal cut-off points of body mass index in Chinese adults. *Biomed Environ Sci*. 2002 Sep;15(3):245-52.

[28] Subramanian S, Strohl KP. A Management Guideline for Obesity-Hypoventilation Syndromes. *Sleep Breath*. 1999;3(4):131-8.

[29] Nowbar S, Burkart KM, Gonzales R, Fedorowicz A, Gozansky WS, Gaudio JC, et al. Obesity-associated hypoventilation in hospitalized patients: prevalence, effects, and outcome. *Am J Med*. 2004 Jan 1;116(1):1-7.

[30] Chiodini I. Clinical review: Diagnosis and treatment of subclinical hypercortisolism. *J Clin Endocrinol Metab*. 2011 May;96(5):1223-36.

[31] Das A, Mukhopadhyay S. The evil axis of obesity, inflammation and type-2 diabetes. *Endocr Metab Immune Disord Drug Targets*. 2011 Mar 1;11(1):23-31.

[32] Duntas LH. Environmental factors and thyroid autoimmunity. *Ann Endocrinol* (Paris). 2011 Apr;72(2):108-13.

[33] Perugini RA, Malkani S. Remission of type 2 diabetes mellitus following bariatric surgery: review of mechanisms and presentation of the concept of 'reversibility'. *Curr Opin Endocrinol Diabetes Obes*. 2011 Apr;18(2):119-28.

[34] Robker RL, Wu LL, Yang X. Inflammatory pathways linking obesity and ovarian dysfunction. *J Reprod Immunol*. 2011 Mar;88(2):142-8.

[35] Spencer SJ, Tilbrook A. The glucocorticoid contribution to obesity. *Stress*. 2011;14(3):233-46.
[36] Teerds KJ, de Rooij DG, Keijer J. Functional relationship between obesity and male reproduction: from humans to animal models. *Hum Reprod Update*. 2011 Sep-Oct;17(5):667-83.
[37] Colditz GA, Willett WC, Rotnitzky A, Manson JE. Weight gain as a risk factor for clinical diabetes mellitus in women. *Ann Intern Med*. 1995 Apr 1;122(7):481-6.
[38] Reaven GM. Relationships among insulin resistance, type 2 diabetes, essential hypertension, and cardiovascular disease: similarities and differences. *J Clin Hypertens* (Greenwich). 2011 Apr;13(4):238-43.
[39] Eckel RH, Kahn SE, Ferrannini E, Goldfine AB, Nathan DM, Schwartz MW, et al. Obesity and type 2 diabetes: what can be unified and what needs to be individualized? *J Clin Endocrinol Metab*. 2011 Jun;96(6):1654-63.
[40] Knowler WC, Barrett-Connor E, Fowler SE, Hamman RF, Lachin JM, Walker EA, et al. Reduction in the incidence of type 2 diabetes with lifestyle intervention or metformin. *N Engl J Med*. 2002 Feb 7;346(6):393-403.
[41] Buchwald H, Estok R, Fahrbach K, Banel D, Jensen MD, Pories WJ, et al. Weight and type 2 diabetes after bariatric surgery: systematic review and meta-analysis. *Am J Med*. 2009 Mar;122(3):248-56 e5.
[42] Taylor EN, Stampfer MJ, Curhan GC. Obesity, weight gain, and the risk of kidney stones. *JAMA*. 2005 Jan 26;293(4):455-62.
[43] Parsons JK. Modifiable risk factors for benign prostatic hyperplasia and lower urinary tract symptoms: new approaches to old problems. *J Urol*. 2007 Aug;178(2):395-401.
[44] Cummings JM, Rodning CB. Urinary stress incontinence among obese women: review of pathophysiology therapy. *Int Urogynecol J Pelvic Floor Dysfunct*. 2000;11(1):41-4.
[45] Hampel H, Abraham NS, El-Serag HB. Meta-analysis: obesity and the risk for gastroesophageal reflux disease and its complications. *Ann Intern Med*. 2005 Aug 2;143(3):199-211.
[46] Cusi K. Role of insulin resistance and lipotoxicity in non-alcoholic steatohepatitis. *Clin Liver Dis*. 2009 Nov;13(4):545-63.
[47] Cusi K. Role of Obesity and Lipotoxicity in the Development of Nonalcoholic Steatohepatitis (Nash): Pathophysiology and Clinical Implications. *Gastroenterology*. 2012 Feb 8.
[48] Stein LL, Dong MH, Loomba R. Insulin sensitizers in nonalcoholic fatty liver disease and steatohepatitis: Current status. *Adv Ther*. 2009 Oct;26(10):893-907.
[49] Weiner RA. Surgical treatment of non-alcoholic steatohepatitis and non-alcoholic fatty liver disease. *Dig Dis*. 2010;28(1):274-9.
[50] Lieverse RJ, Jansen JB, Masclee AA, Lamers CB. Gastrointestinal disturbances with obesity. *Scand J Gastroenterol Suppl*. 1993;200:53-8.
[51] Erlinger S. Gallstones in obesity and weight loss. *Eur J Gastroenterol Hepatol*. 2000 Dec;12(12):1347-52.
[52] Faloon WW. Hepatobiliary effects of obesity and weight-reducing surgery. *Semin Liver Dis*. 1988 Aug;8(3):229-36.
[53] Weinsier RL, Ullmann DO. Gallstone formation and weight loss. *Obes Res*. 1993 Jan;1(1):51-6.

[54] Hitt HC, McMillen RC, Thornton-Neaves T, Koch K, Cosby AG. Comorbidity of obesity and pain in a general population: results from the Southern Pain Prevalence Study. *J Pain*. 2007 May;8(5):430-6.

[55] Zettel-Watson L, Rutledge DN, Aquino JK, Cantero P, Espinoza A, Leal F, et al. Typology of chronic pain among overweight Mexican Americans. *J Health Care Poor Underserved*. 2011 Aug;22(3):1030-47.

[56] Anandacoomarasamy A, Caterson I, Sambrook P, Fransen M, March L. The impact of obesity on the musculoskeletal system. *Int J Obes* (Lond). 2008 Feb;32(2):211-22.

[57] Tuzun EH. Quality of life in chronic musculoskeletal pain. *Best Pract Res Clin Rheumatol*. 2007 Jun;21(3):567-79.

[58] Wearing SC, Hennig EM, Byrne NM, Steele JR, Hills AP. Musculoskeletal disorders associated with obesity: a biomechanical perspective. *Obes Rev*. 2006 Aug;7(3):239-50.

[59] Anandacoomarasamy A, Fransen M, March L. Obesity and the musculoskeletal system. *Curr Opin Rheumatol*. 2009 Jan;21(1):71-7.

[60] Chan G, Chen CT. Musculoskeletal effects of obesity. *Curr Opin Pediatr*. 2009 Feb;21(1):65-70.

[61] Behrens C, Tang BQ, Amson BJ. Early results of a Canadian laparoscopic sleeve gastrectomy experience. *Can J Surg*. 2011 Apr;54(2):138-43.

[62] Brancatisano A, Wahlroos S, Brancatisano R. Improvement in comorbid illness after placement of the Swedish Adjustable Gastric Band. *Surg Obes Relat Dis*. 2008 May-Jun;4(3 Suppl):S39-46.

[63] Allison DB, Fontaine KR, Manson JE, Stevens J, VanItallie TB. Annual deaths attributable to obesity in the United States. *JAMA*. 1999 Oct 27;282(16):1530-8.

[64] Calle EE, Rodriguez C, Walker-Thurmond K, Thun MJ. Overweight, obesity, and mortality from cancer in a prospectively studied cohort of U.S. adults. *N Engl J Med*. 2003 Apr 24;348(17):1625-38.

[65] Ligibel J. Obesity and breast cancer. *Oncology* (Williston Park). 2011 Oct;25(11):994-1000.

[66] Morimoto LM, White E, Chen Z, Chlebowski RT, Hays J, Kuller L, et al. Obesity, body size, and risk of postmenopausal breast cancer: the Women's Health Initiative (United States). *Cancer Causes Control*. 2002 Oct;13(8):741-51.

[67] Chlebowski RT, Aiello E, McTiernan A. Weight loss in breast cancer patient management. *J Clin Oncol*. 2002 Feb 15;20(4):1128-43.

[68] Cleary MP, Maihle NJ. The role of body mass index in the relative risk of developing premenopausal versus postmenopausal breast cancer. *Proc Soc Exp Biol Med*. 1997 Oct;216(1):28-43.

[69] Carmichael AR. Obesity and prognosis of breast cancer. *Obes Rev*. 2006 Nov;7(4):333-40.

[70] Moghaddam AA, Woodward M, Huxley R. Obesity and risk of colorectal cancer: a meta-analysis of 31 studies with 70,000 events. *Cancer Epidemiol Biomarkers Prev*. 2007 Dec;16(12):2533-47.

[71] Li D, Morris JS, Liu J, Hassan MM, Day RS, Bondy ML, et al. Body mass index and risk, age of onset, and survival in patients with pancreatic cancer. *JAMA*. 2009 Jun 24;301(24):2553-62.

[72] Garcia Hidalgo L. Dermatological complications of obesity. *Am J Clin Dermatol*. 2002;3(7):497-506.

[73] Hahler B. An overview of dermatological conditions commonly associated with the obese patient. *Ostomy Wound Manage*. 2006 Jun;52(6):34-6, 8, 40 passim.
[74] Mathur AN, Goebel L. Skin findings associated with obesity. *Adolesc Med State Art Rev*. 2011 Apr;22(1):146-56, ix.
[75] Scheinfeld NS. Obesity and dermatology. *Clin Dermatol*. 2004 Jul-Aug;22(4):303-9.
[76] Shipman AR, Millington GW. Obesity and the skin. *Br J Dermatol*. 2011 Oct;165(4):743-50.
[77] van Hout GC, van Oudheusden I, van Heck GL. Psychological profile of the morbidly obese. *Obes Surg*. 2004 May;14(5):579-88.
[78] Fabricatore AN, Wadden TA. Psychological aspects of obesity. *Clin Dermatol*. 2004 Jul-Aug;22(4):332-7.
[79] Black DW, Goldstein RB, Mason EE. Psychiatric diagnosis and weight loss following gastric surgery for obesity. *Obes Surg*. 2003 Oct;13(5):746-51.
[80] Charles SC. Psychiatric evaluation of morbidly obese patients. *Gastroenterol Clin North Am*. 1987 Sep;16(3):415-32.
[81] Foster GD, Sarwer DB, Wadden TA. Psychological effects of weight cycling in obese persons: a review and research agenda. *Obes Res*. 1997 Sep;5(5):474-88.
[82] [Sikorski C, Luppa M, Kaiser M, Glaesmer H, Schomerus G, Konig HH, et al. The stigma of obesity in the general public and its implications for public health - a systematic review. *BMC Public Health*. 2011;11:661.
[83] Guh DP, Zhang W, Bansback N, Amarsi Z, Birmingham CL, Anis AH. The incidence of co-morbidities related to obesity and overweight: a systematic review and meta-analysis. *BMC Public Health*. 2009;9:88.

Section 2: The Preoperative Management of the Bariatric Patient

In: The Fundamentals of Bariatric Surgery
Editors: Shahzeer Karmali and Daniel W. Birch
ISBN: 978-1-62417-732-3

Chapter 3

Nutrition Assessment of the Bariatric Patient: Pre-operative

Carlene Johnson Stoklossa and Janet Stadnyk
Nutrition Services, Alberta Health ServicesEdmonton, AB, Canada

Abstract

This chapter provides an overview of the key components of an adult obesity nutrition assessment. Nutrition assessment by a registered dietitian is recommended prior to bariatric surgery, as part of a comprehensive weight management treatment plan. Treatment for morbid obesity, including bariatric surgery, is more successful when multidisciplinary health care providers assess, treat, monitor and evaluate individuals both before and after surgery.

All patients should have a comprehensive food and nutrition history that considers food and nutrient intake, nutrition-related knowledge and practices, food availability, barriers to change, self-monitoring, self management practices, and physical activity. The nutrition assessment should include a review of relevant data to identify conditions either associated with or contributing to obesity. Analysis and interpretation of relevant data should be made using reference standards to identify abnormal values and direct appropriate diagnosis and intervention strategies. Clinical practice guidelines for obesity [1] as well as co-morbid diseases (e.g. diabetes [2], hypertension) should be considered when creating care plans.

Bariatric surgery has a significant impact on nutritional status. Biochemical assessment is recommended to assess for possible vitamin and mineral deficiencies prior to bariatric surgery. Key components of nutrition interventions and education provided in preparation for bariatric surgery are discussed.

Introduction

Obesity is a chronic disease that impacts a patient's physical, social and mental health. Patients with obesity should have a comprehensive nutrition assessment completed by a registered dietitian to identify any nutrition-related problems and their causes. The organization and terminology used in this chapter is consistent with standardized language and nutrition care process [3]. A patient's history is reviewed to identify acute or chronic illnesses that have nutritional implications. A thorough history also includes behavioural components such as readiness for change, realistic goal setting and general knowledge of nutrition. A multi-factorial approach to determine the nutritional status of an individual is recommended and is reviewed below.

- A comprehensive patient history is needed to identify information relevant to obesity and co-morbid conditions.
- Personal and family/social history is important to review as it may identify potential barriers to better target the nutrition intervention.
- A detailed weight history is needed to provide a thorough overview of weight status and changes throughout the person's lifetime. Measurement of height and weight is completed.
- A review of past weight management interventions should include all methods used to control weight with details on when it was tried, number of attempts and impact on weight.
- A review of expectations of treatment including weight outcomes
- Readiness to change is an important factor to determine whether and when to initiate treatment and the success of treatment. Methods to assess readiness may include Stage of Change, current life stressors, support systems, reasons to lose weight, maintain weight or prevent weight gain at this time, expectations of treatment and weight management goals.
- Medical and surgical history should focus on identification of possible causes and complications of obesity and obesity-related disorders. Severity of obesity, limitations and extent of disability should be evaluated as well.
- A mental health history may be able to identify psychological factors contributing to weight gain or potential barriers to treatment.
- A review of knowledge and understanding of the nutritional impact of interventions for obesity, including bariatric surgery.

Based on a comprehensive nutrition assessment and information gathered as part of follow up care, the registered dietitian can assist the team with overall treatment plans. There are four key objectives of nutrition intervention prior to bariatric surgery [4].

1) Improve nutritional status
2) Improve control of nutrition-related co-morbidities
3) Improve or develop lifestyle habits that promote positive health outcomes after bariatric surgery
4) Educate the patient about the nutritional impact of bariatric surgery

Monitoring and evaluation is a process of reviewing the patient progress and relevant data to compare with the intervention plan. Adjustments or modifications to the care plan are made with attention give to identifying and managing barriers that are preventing the patient from reaching identified goals.

Nutrition Assessment

Personal and Family/Social History

Personal history includes information regarding a patient's occupation including occupation status, hours of work, work environment, support services (e.g. employee assistance programs), disability, retirement and previous work experience. Education and language (e.g. verbal and written skills) and comprehension are very important to assess.

Family/social history includes information on a patient's housing situation, household members, role in the family, socioeconomic status, cultural and religious beliefs and social isolation/connection. The weight and health history of family members may also provide information regarding risk of co-morbid conditions. Information on family dynamics related to food and eating, the role of food in the person's life and culture/religion and their parenting style (e.g. use of food as a reward). Environment has a significant impact on lifestyle choices and the ability to implement and sustain changes. Information regarding a patient's work, home and social networks are important to identify potential barriers and target nutrition interventions.

Weight History

A detailed weight history is important to assess the potential causes of obesity and target interventions. Weight can be a sensitive topic to discuss for many people. Suggestions for terminology and sample questions have been provided to assist health care providers with obtaining a detailed history in a respectful manner. **(See Table 1)** Both measurement and discussion of weight should be conducted in private (e.g. in a counselling room) rather than a public area (e.g. waiting room or hallway). Obesity is a chronic disease with a typical pattern of slow progressive gain over time. Weight stability can be defined as a change of ± 2% from either baseline weight (loss phase) or current weight (maintenance phase). Prevention of gain (maintenance) is an important clinical outcome and should not be viewed as a lack of result.

Table 1. Detailed Weight History

Data	Background and Key Questions
Measure current weight	Key Questions As part of our session, I would like to measure your weight today. Is this ok with you? Would you prefer to do this at the start of our session or at the end?
	Note: It may be beneficial to measure weight at the beginning of the session. Many patients are too preoccupied to focus on the discussion if they are weighed at the end of
	Note: It may be beneficial to measure weight at the beginning of the session. Many patients are too preoccupied to focus on the discussion if they are weighed at the end of

Table 1. (Continued)

Data	Background and Key Questions
Determine weight ranges	Is your weight today your highest weight? Can you share with me your highest weight? When was this (year, age)? What was your lowest weight as an adult? Was there a time when your weight was stable for more than 6 months? What was that weight?
Determine weight status between age of onset and today	Have there been any changes in your weight in the past 6 months? Compared to today, what was your weight one year ago? 5 years ago? Can you remember your weight in grade school? teens? 20's? 30's? 40's? 50's?
Determine age of onset of excess weight. Life stages that may be associated with significant changes in weight include preschool (before age 5), pre-pubertal, adolescence and adulthood.	At what point in your life was weight a concern for you? When would you say that you noticed you were significantly heavier than others? (e.g. schoolmates, friends, family, colleagues)
Explore relationship between weight and major life events.	What changes to health, if any, have you experienced that have affected your weight? (e.g. changes due to illness or injury, pregnancy) Can you share with me any major life event or change in life stage that has impacted your weight? (e.g. transitions from high-school to university, school to work, single to married, move from family home to on their own, becoming a parent)
Explore pattern of weight changes	Most patients tell us there are two common weight change patterns. A "yo-yo" pattern, with significant decreases and increases in weight or a pattern of "slow but steady" gain over time. Can you share with me what your pattern is?

Weight Control and Intervention History

Patients seeking treatment for obesity may have tried different methods of weight control in the past. Documentation of each method tried including the length of intervention, changes in weight and the costs/benefits of the interventions as seen by the patient are important to understand patient experience and knowledge. Questionnaires can be used to obtain the history in a quick and comprehensive manner. Both recommended and non-recommended weight control methods should be documented, including interventions that may require further investigation such as eating disorder behaviours, substance abuse or harmful interventions that may require medical assessment. Medication, herbal and supplement history should also be reviewed to determine impact on weight status and evaluate previous interventions for weight management.

Weight Goals and Expectations

Patients often set a goal weight based upon height/weight reference tables or a self-defined ideal weight [5]. There is a considerable gap between patient expectations to lose more than 30% of their body weight with treatment outcomes of 10 to 20% [6]. One study found both goal (amount of weight expected to lose in a program) and ideal (how much they would like to weigh) weights are unrealistically high for both men and women [7]. Unrealistic weight outcomes are common, with a higher frequency in younger patients, patients who attribute their obesity to physical causes and do not attribute it to behavioural ones. It is important to assess weight goals and treatment expectations. Unrealistic goals are correlated with false hopes, lower satisfaction, reduced motivation, higher attrition, poor weight loss outcomes and poor long-term maintenance of weight loss [6].

Knowledge, Beliefs and Attitudes [8]

There are many misconceptions about nutrition, activity and weight management. Source of nutrition information for patients may be friends, family, the media, or the diet industry. Patients may be resistant or anxious about seeing a registered dietitian. Long histories of weight loss attempts may mean patients feel they "know it all already", "do not want to be told what to do" or they think they will "have to give up their favourite foods". It can be challenging for people to record their food/beverage intake and activity for evaluation as they may feel embarrassed or judged. It is important to assess the beliefs and attitudes of the patient towards weight management and health care providers in order to establish a positive working relationship.

Explaining your role and developing a partnership with the patient can help them determine and achieve their goals. Health care professionals need to recognize that their own knowledge, beliefs and attitudes towards obesity may also impact the care provided. Patients who are seeking treatment for obesity have tried multiple methods of weight loss in the past. To assess their knowledge and beliefs about nutrition, health care providers should evaluate any misconceptions regarding diet/nutrition and weight or food restriction or avoidance and document any diets the patient has attempted or is currently following.

Attitudes towards food (e.g. good vs. bad food, banned foods) and toward lifestyle change are important to understand. As well, it is important to assess their understanding of nutrition concepts, as many patients require re-education regarding nutrition facts and dieting myths.

Although people may be overweight or obese, they may not be ready, willing or able to implement lifestyle changes at this time. Determining the stage of change or readiness for change will help to decide if intervention for weight management should be initiated and identify the degree of weight management readiness and importance to the patient. A patient's motivation and the reasons to pursue treatment, including outcome expectations, should be documented. Barriers to activity, nutrition, behaviour modification or self management should be assessed, with referral to other health care providers as needed. Some people may have low acceptance of new foods or are not willing to try new foods, which is a barrier to making changes to their intake. Low self-efficacy, negative self talk and rigid cognitive constructs (e.g. all-or-nothing thinking) may also be barriers to successful treatment and require assessment and coordination of care with mental health professionals.

Food and Nutrient Intake [8, 9]

Assessment of both quantity and quality of food and nutrient intake should be detailed for weight management intervention. It is important to determine intake from all sources (food, beverages and supplements) to determine total energy intake. Meal and snack patterns should also be noted as these may help identify frequency and adequacy of overall intake.

Macronutrient intake should be assessed to determine if both percentage and total grams of carbohydrate, fat, protein and fibre are within recommendations. Intake of beverages, including milk, juice, pop, caffeinated beverages and alcohol should be assessed not only for their caloric content but for their nutrient, fluid and other bioactive substance content. Adequate caloric intake does not guarantee adequate micronutrient intake; deficiencies can occur even with adequate calories. For example, despite very high caloric intakes there is a higher incidence of vitamin D deficiency in people with obesity. Women in weight management programs, many of whom are in child-bearing years, should have calcium, vitamin D, iron and folic acid status assessed.

A complete diet history should include previous methods or treatments used for weight management. The assessment should also include details on the person's access to food, grocery shopping, meal preparation and eating out. Environment (location, atmosphere, alone or with company) is one of the biggest influences on food choices and intake and can help identify important influences to eating behaviour and food selection. The reasons and influences for food choices including hunger, cravings and trigger foods should be part of the assessment as well.

Factors Affecting Access to Food

Food Availability

The availability of healthy and safe food and food/nutrition related supplies directly impacts intake. Factors affecting access are numerous. It is a misconception that someone who is obese has an adequate supply of food. They may have adequate calories to support a higher body weight, but the quality of their food intake may be poor. Access to quality food, proper equipment for preparation and storage and ability to make safe and healthy choices are important aspects of a nutrition assessment.

All sources of food, including groceries, restaurants, food banks, food from family and friends, food at work or schools should be assessed.

Mobility

People may have barriers to achieve their nutrition-related activities of daily living. Limited mobility can impact ability to purchase and transport food to one's home. It can also impact the ability to prepare foods, thereby increasing the frequency of eating convenience foods or restaurant/take-out meals. Some people may rely on friends and family to assist them with shopping and food preparation, which may impact the choices available. Social support to make healthy choices is important and may present as a barrier if others in the person's environment are not supportive.

Knowledge

A lack of knowledge on meal planning and preparation, label reading or eating on a budget may impact healthy food choices at home, at the grocery store or when eating out. Lack of planning or lack of time/time management may influence people to choose more convenience foods or restaurant/take-out meals.

Finances

Limited finances can restrict the intake of fresh fruits and vegetables. Low cost foods or "meal deals" are often calorie-dense but nutrient-poor foods. People may be able to obtain adequate supplies after receiving payment from work or support services, but as finances are depleted, their access to food becomes more limited. For some people, a "feast/famine" cycle can develop, resulting in overeating when money is available and inadequate intake as funds become limited. Information regarding how to eat healthy on a limited budget may address barriers or perceptions that, although difficult, it is achievable.

Behaviour

Self-monitoring and self-management practices are two key behaviours that are important to the management of chronic disease. Self monitoring tools may include a daily journal, body weight scale, glucometer or blood pressure monitor, tools to measure food portions (e.g. measuring cups/spoons, kitchen scale) and reliable references for nutrition/calories (e.g. food labels, websites, books or reference tables such as the Nutrient Value of Some Common Foods[10]).

Assessment of behaviour should include the actions and activities that influence the achievement of the individual's goal. Attendance at appointments and use of self-monitoring tools can be measures to determine adherence. Assessment of mealtime behaviours should include meal duration (e.g. eating slow or fast, taking time for a break or working though lunch) and focus of attention (e.g. focusing on enjoying the meal or eating while distracted). Questions should be asked to assess the patient's ability to recall education provided and compliance with previous instruction. Maladaptive behaviours such as avoidance, impulsivity, lack of ability to delay gratification, sabotage, emotional eating, binge eating, and binge/purge should be assessed; referral to mental health providers may be required.

Medical and Surgical History

Past or current medical and/or surgical history should be evaluated for its impact on the nutrition care of the patient. The following provides an overview of certain medical conditions and surgical procedures and their relationship to nutrition and weight management.

Medications and Herbal Supplements

It is important to assess all medication and supplement use to determine their impact on nutritional status and weight. People with obesity may be on medications for other medical conditions that can impact weight or appetite. As with all patients, nutrient/food-medication interactions need to be evaluated.

With the high percentage of people seeking methods to treat obesity, many products are available on the market that target weight management. Most have limited or no benefit; others may cause harm. Evidence for the efficacy of a dietary supplement to stimulate weight loss is often absent or inconclusive [11]. In many cases, there is insufficient evidence to recommend in favour for or against the use of herbal remedies, dietary supplements or homeopathic medicines for weight management in the obese person [11]. Safety concerns arise due to the lack of adequate labelling or evaluation from a regulatory body on these products. There is also the risk of possible drug-nutrient interactions [11].

Cardiovascular and Respiratory Health

There are a number of reasons for weight fluctuations related to cardiovascular and respiratory health that should be evaluated. For example, some medications such as betablockers can decrease heart rate influencing metabolic rate and the ability to manage weight. Weight changes may also be a result of fluid shifts due to cardiac insufficiency or poor cardiorespiratory status which limits exercise tolerance and decreases energy expenditure. Respiratory disorders that are common in obesity include obstructive sleep apnea, chronic obstructive pulmonary disease (COPD), asthma and obesity hypoventilation syndrome. Smoking cessation can also impact weight and is commonly associated with a weight gain of up to 7 kg. Patient history should include details on smoking (e.g. amount, frequency, start date, and stop date if they have quit smoking).

Endocrine Disorders

Several endocrine disorders (e.g. polycystic ovarian syndrome, hypothyroidism, Cushing's syndrome) impact hormone levels involved in the regulation of metabolic rate or utilization of substrate. Weight gain and alterations to body composition (e.g. increase in body fat percentage) may result if untreated. Vitamin B 12 deficiencies are more common in patients taking medications such as Metformin.

Reproductive Health

Obesity can impair the fertility of both men and women. However, weight loss can produce hormone changes associated with improved fertility. For women who have had children, it is important to assess the weight changes associated with each pregnancy. Pre-pregnant weight, weight change during pregnancy, birth weight, and maternal weight changes after the birth should be documented as part of their weight history.

Women are at a higher risk of obesity if they do not return to their baseline weight by 6 months post-partum. Some women have experienced significant weight gain with pregnancy (e.g. > 16 kg), contributing to obesity. Women with mennorhagia may be at increased risk of iron deficiency anemia.

Gastrointestinal Disorders

Gastrointestinal disorders common to obesity (e.g. gastroesophageal reflux disease, hernias) may impact nutritional status and food selection. Non-alcoholic fatty liver disease (NAFLD) is common in people with obesity and may **not** cause alterations in liver enzymes. Weight loss may be required to improve liver treatment outcomes (e.g. transplant). People with renal disease may experience fluid shifts that impact weight status. Weight loss may be recommended to improve renal treatment outcomes (e.g. transplant, dialysis).

Muscular-Skeletal/Neurological Impairments

Muscular-skeletal and/or neurological concerns may limit mobility and exercise tolerance, thereby decreasing energy expenditure. It is not uncommon for individuals with obesity to have orthopedic injuries or surgeries related to the spine or joints, affecting mobility.

Chronic pain associated with muscular-skeletal and/or neurological problems may also impair one's ability to perform activities of daily life including shopping, cooking, eating and activity. In addition, the medications to treat pain may cause constipation and decreased appetite. Cognitive impairments may impact an individual's ability to read or write, communicate, learn, remember or understand instructions, presenting significant barriers to implement behaviour change.

Mental Health

Mental health disorders, especially if undiagnosed or untreated, may present a significant barrier to obesity management. Several mental health diagnoses and related medications can impact a patient's level of alertness and cause changes in taste, mouth care (dry mouth), appetite, bowel function and weight. Depending on the diagnosis and status, individuals may have an impaired ability to understand instructions and/or implement behaviour change. A referral for treatment of mental health concerns prior to aggressive treatment and active participation in a weight management program may be indicated.

Table 2. Binge Eating Disorder [12]

Binge eating disorder (BED) is a psychiatric disorder in which a subject shows the following symptoms:
Periodically does not exercise control over consumption of food. Eats an unusually large amount of food at one time -- more than a normal person would eat in the same amount of time. Eats much more quickly during binge episodes than during normal eating episodes. Eats until physically uncomfortable. Eats large amounts of food even when they are not really hungry. Usually eats alone during binge eating episodes, in order to avoid discovery of the disorder. Often eats alone during periods of normal eating, owing to feelings of embarrassment about food. Feels disgusted, depressed or guilty after binge eating.
The formal diagnosis criteria are similar in that subjects must **binge at least twice per week for a minimum period of three months.** Unlike in bulimia, those with BED do not purge, fast or engage in strenuous exercise after binge eating. BED is similar to, but is distinct from, compulsive overeating. Those with BED do not have a compulsion to overeat and do not spend a great deal of time fantasizing about food. On the contrary, some people with binge eating disorder have very negative feelings about food. Currently, the **DSM IV-TR** categorizes this cluster of behaviours or symptoms under "Eating Disorder Not Otherwise Specified (EDNOS)".

Patients and health care providers commonly use the word "binge" or "compulsive" to describe a number of different eating behaviours. Detailed questions are important to document the event, including the type and amount of food eaten, the rate of eating and the person's response after the event (e.g. feelings, actions, restrictions, etc). This information will help to determine if the event is within a normal range of behaviour (e.g. eating two cookies when they are hot out of the oven instead of one), related to portion control (e.g. eating large amounts without a loss of control or inappropriate responses after the event), or if the behaviour is consistent with a diagnosis of an eating disorder.

A summary of the diagnosis for binge eating disorder [12] is provided for reference only (see Table 2). An assessment by a mental health specialist is required to make a diagnosis and determine appropriate treatment. The focus of treatment for people with new or unstable mental health diagnoses should be to stabilize the mental health concern and minimize nutritional impact or risk. Some individuals may not be appropriate for weight loss or obesity treatment at the time, but may be appropriate for nutrition intervention. Coordination of nutrition care with appropriate referrals is recommended.

Biochemical Data [1]

Biochemical data should be reviewed with relevant data included as part of the nutrition assessment to identify information relevant to obesity and co-morbid conditions **(see Table 3)** [8]. Blood work is required to screen for possible vitamin and mineral deficiencies that are more common in obesity or may be impacted by treatment options (e.g. medication or bariatric surgery). Micronutrients of concern in bariatric surgery include calcium, vitamin D, iron, vitamin B12 and folic acid [4]. Biochemical monitoring is recommended before and after bariatric surgery as part of a comprehensive nutrition care plan [13].

Table 3. Biochemical Data

Category	Biochemical data
Electrolyte and renal	sodium, potassium, chloride, magnesium, phosphorus, parathyroid hormone (PTH), creatinine, urea, serum calcium, GFR, BUN
Endocrine	serum glucose (fasting, random, 2 hr PC), HbA1C, glucose tolerance test thyroid function (TSH, T3, T4), fasting insulin, testosterone
Category	**Biochemical data**
Gastrointestinal	alkaline phosphatase, AST, ALT, GGT, bilirubin, amylase
Lipid Profile	total cholesterol, triglyceride, LDL, HDL, Ratio total cholesterol: HDL
Nutritional anemia	complete blood count (CBC) with differential, serum iron, ferritin, total iron-binding capacity (TIBC), serum RBC folate or plasma homocysteine, vitamin B12, PTT, INR
Protein	albumin, prealbumin, total serum protein, transferrin
Urinalysis	Colour, osmolality, USG, volume, ketones, glucose, protein
Vitamins and minerals	iron, ferritin, calcium , 25-OH vitamin D, vitamin B12, RBC folate, thiamin

Vitamin D and Obesity

BMI is inversely associated with serum vitamin D concentrations, with patients who have a BMI>30 kg/m^2 having the lowest levels [14]. Prior to gastric bypass surgery, one study found 80% of obese subjects to have 25-OH vitamin D levels below 32 ng/mL (80 nmol/L) [15]. The relationship persists even when other factors are controlled such as sun exposure and nutrient intake from diet or supplements [16]. The exact mechanism is unknown [17]. Factors such as social isolation and stigmatization, mobility limitations and concern about risk of falls may contribute to further reduce outdoor UV exposure. It is possible the fat soluble vitamin may be held in the adipose tissue with slower or impaired mobilization to the serum [18]. However, a decrease in adipose tissue with weight loss does not increase the bioavailability of vitamin D [17] and deficiencies persist after gastric bypass without supplementation [19]. Other research suggests decreased bioavailability of the skin-derived source of the vitamin [20]. Further research is warranted.

Although the main source of vitamin D is the sun [30], little vitamin D is produced by the skin in the winter or at times other than solar noon, even in the summer [21]. Most Canadians do not get adequate UVR with summer exposure to maintain levels throughout the year. The highest prevalence of deficiency occurred from October to March [17, 21]. Use of sunscreen with an SPF of $\geq$8 reduces the amount of vitamin D produced by the skin by 95%. [22] People who live in northern climates (above 40°N), use sunscreen, are overweight, have limited exposure to the sun, have darker skin, or who are over 50 years old [17] need more vitamin D [23].

Monitoring and Evaluation

Serum vitamin D (25-OH D) is the best indicator or the nutritional and functional status of vitamin D [30]. It reflects the adequacy of vitamin D from skin production, diet and supplementation. Serum 25-OH vitamin D levels do not indicate the amount of vitamin D stored in other body tissues [23]. Serum levels should be completed in August/September to assess peak summer values (greatest sun exposure) and February/March for peak winter values (least sun exposure). As the half life of 25-OH vitamin D is 15-20 days, monitoring of serum values are recommended no sooner than 3 months after start of supplementation [30]. Individuals taking supplements about the upper tolerable level (UL= 2000 IU) should have monitoring of serum values.

Current best practice recommendations include monitoring serum levels to achieve and maintain vitamin D above 75 nmol/L [23]. It is unknown if different serum concentrations are required for different clinical outcomes, including prevention of deficiency, adequacy for bone health and optimal levels for health promotion and disease prevention.

Requirements

Most Canadians require supplementation to achieve 25-OH vitamin D levels >75 nmol/L [14].

- Low risk adults under 50 year of age are recommended to take 400-1000 IU daily.
- Higher doses are required for high-risk and older adults
- Doses up to 2000IU are safe and do not require monitoring
- If higher doses are needed, monitoring is appropriate

Requirements are higher with obesity. Specific recommendations for people with obesity or bariatric surgery have yet to be determined. Daily requirements as indicated by the DRI [24], or other health care bodies (Health Canada [25] Osteoporosis Society of Canada [30]) may underestimate needs for this population. Daily intakes of 5000 IU may be required for obese adults to maintain normal serum levels throughout the year, especially at northern latitudes [14, 20,26, 30].

The majority of patients in weight management or bariatric surgery programs are women of reproductive age. Serum vitamin D levels of infants correlate with maternal serum vitamin

D, therefore babies born to or breast fed by deficient mothers should also be considered deficient.

Supplementation

Supplements are commonly available in two strengths, 400 IU or 1000 IU, in either tablet or liquid (mL or drops). Vitamin D may be included as an ingredient in some vitamin or calcium supplements. There are two forms of vitamin D: Vitamin D3 (cholecalciferol) and Vitamin D2 (ergocalciferol). D2 is plant derived and requires conversion to Vitamin D3. Research is conflicting whether D2 supplements are as effective as D3. For high dose therapies (50 000 IU), vitamin D3 is almost twice as effective at raising 25(OH) vitamin D levels than D2 [27] and was more effective at maintaining serum levels [28]. Other studies using lower daily doses (1000 IU) found both forms were effective at maintaining vitamin D status [29]. Further research is warranted.

Treatment of Deficiency

Current treatment for vitamin D deficiency recommends using vitamin D3 (cholecalciferol) supplements. An increase of 1 mcg (40 IU) of vitamin D3 can increase the serum by 1 mmol/L [17, 26, 29, 30]. In general, daily intakes of approximately 1700 IU vitamin D3 are needed to raise serum concentrations from 50 to 80 nmol/L [17]. Short term high dose supplementation ("Stoss" or "push" therapy) may be indicated to treat severe (<25 nmol/L) vitamin D deficiencies. This treatment provides 50 000IU vitamin D each week for 8 weeks (e.g. take 7 of the 1000 IU pills daily for 8 weeks) [14, 26]. Bloodwork should be completed at the end of this treatment to assess biochemical response and inform supplementation dose. For any level of deficiency, people with obesity and vitamin D deficiency need treatment for 8 to 12 weeks [17, 31]. and may need higher daily doses up to 5000 IU vitamin D3 to maintain normal serum levels [26]. Serum levels should be monitored every 3 months until normal levels are achieved.

Vitamin D Excess and Toxicity

Serum 25 OH Vitamin D levels of > 200 nmol/L are excessive and >350 nmol/L are toxic. Health risks of excess vitamin D include nausea, vomiting, poor appetite, constipation, weakness, weight loss, elevated serum calcium, confusion, deposit of calcium into tissues, kidney damage and heart rhythm abnormalities. Vitamin D toxicity can result from excessive intake for a prolonged period of time. Case reports of toxicity have been documented with use of supplements that contain extremely high doses (e.g. Soladek 600,000 IU Vitamin D, 120,000 IU vitamin A and 5 mg vitamin E) [32]. Short term high dose supplementation (50 000 IU per week for 8 weeks) or excess sun exposure has not caused toxicity [33].

Assessing Energy Requirements

Resting Energy Expenditure

An accurate assessment of energy needs is required in developing a nutrition care plan. Resting metabolic rate (RMR), also known as resting energy expenditure (REE), is the largest single component of total daily caloric expenditure. Indirect calorimetry is considered the "gold" standard method of determining RMR and should be used, if available, as predictive equations will be less accurate [34].

Various predictive equations have been developed to estimate RMR. The accuracy rate of all predictive equations decreases with obese versus non-obese adults [35]. The common clinical practice of using an adjusted body weight to estimate the metabolically active tissue mass does not improve the accuracy of predicting metabolic rate in obese individuals and is not supported by evidence [35, 36]. Both fat-free mass and fat mass contribute to RMR. However, there is no fixed value to estimate the percentage of fat mass that is metabolically active and contributes to total energy expenditure [36].

The **Mifflin-St. Jeor** [37] equation has been validated for use in overweight and obese adults using actual body weight. It has been found to be the most accurate estimate of RMR with at least 70% accuracy, with acceptable errors of underestimation (up to 20%) and minimal overestimation errors (up to 15%) of measured RMR.

Male: RMR = [9.99 x weight (kg)] + [6.25 x height (cm)] – [4.92 x age (years)] + 5
FemaleRMR = [9.99 x weight (kg)] + [6.25 x height (cm)] – [4.92 x age (years)] - 161

Total Energy Expenditure

The energy consumed by physical activity needs to be added to the REE to determine the total energy expenditure. Energy expended from activity is the most variable component (ranging from less than 10% for people who are immobile to more than 50% for athletes) of total energy requirements and is difficult to determine accurately. People of higher weights burn more calories for a specific activity compared to a lower weight person, as they are required to move more body weight to perform that activity. However, the ratio or relationship is variable and has not been determined. Energy expenditure tables are available [38], however health care professionals should use with caution as there is limited research to measure the energy expenditure from activity for people with higher BMI.

Baseline activity level should be assessed and used to compare against reference standards and as a comparison for change. A daily average of energy expenditure can be calculated by assessing the frequency, intensity, type and duration of each activity. If the level of activity does not exceed 150 minutes of moderate intensity activity per week, the energy expenditure is not sufficient to produce significant changes in weight to require caloric adjustment. The recommended physical activity (PA) coefficient is summarized in **Table 4**. No adjustment to the REE (e.g. use PA = 1.0) is needed to account for this level of physical activity [39].

Table 4. Physical Activity Coefficient (PA) for Different Activity Levels [38, 40 41]

Activity Level	Description	Energy Expenditure	PA
sedentary	Only activities of daily life, no planned or intentional activity	<5000 steps/day	1.00
low active	Activities of daily life and planned activities of mostly low intensity; e.g., walking 1.5-3 miles/day at 3-4 mph	5000- 7499 steps/day or <1000 kcal/week	1.00
moderate active	Activities of daily life and planned activities including some moderate intensity; e.g., walking >3 miles/day at 3-4 mph	7500-9999 steps/day, 150kcal/day or 1000 to <2500 kcal/week	1.12
high active	Activities of daily life and planned activities including vigorous intensity levels	≥10000 steps/day or 2250-3500 kcal/week	1.27
very high active	Activities of daily life and planned activities including vigorous intensity levels	>15000 steps/day or >3500 kcal/ week	1.45

Nutrition Prescription

The nutrition prescription is the individualized recommended intake of energy, foods and nutrients. Therapeutic targets for nutrition intervention for adults with overweight and obesity should primarily target energy intake to assist with weight loss and prevention of weight re-gain.

As overweight and obesity are independent risk factors for other chronic disease, the nutrition prescription should be consistent with standards for nutrition adequacy (e.g. Dietary Reference Intakes [DRI] and Acceptable Macronutrient Distribution Ranges [AMDR]). The prescription should not be below the DRI (at least the Recommended Dietary Allowances [RDA] or Adequate Intake [AI] amounts) and meet the standards for the specific disease or condition. Clinical practice guidelines have been established for several conditions including cardio-protective guidelines (e.g. cardiovascular disease [42], diabetes [2], dyslipidemia [49]) and osteoporosis [30]. Health care providers should also refer to the individual guidelines for specific co-morbid conditions. There are some differences in recommendations depending on the disease state or guideline. A summary of nutrition components for weight management and cardio-protective guidelines can be found in **Table 5.** For nutrition prescription and goals after bariatric surgery **see Chapter 14.**

Total Energy

Assessment of total daily energy requirements includes resting energy requirements (measured or estimated) and physical activity level. Resting energy requirements should be measured via indirect calorimetry [8, 9, 35]. If a predictive equation is used, it is recommended to use the Mifflin-St. Jeor equation [24] and actual body weight. To produce an average weight loss of 0.5-1 kg (1-2 pounds) per week requires a deficit of 500-1000 kcal per day from total estimated energy needs [8]. Energy expenditure is variable and difficult to measure or estimate. No adjustment or coefficient is required to account for energy expenditure unless physical activity is greater than 150 minutes of moderate intensity activity per week. A practical way to achieve this deficit is to subtract 500 kcal from resting energy requirements. This method is usually sufficient to produce a 500-1000kcal deficit from total energy requirements, resulting in weight loss.

Total caloric intake should not be lower than 1200 kcal without physician supervision. Very-low-calorie diets (VLCD) that provide ≤800 calories per day must be prescribed by a physician [8]. Individuals must be monitored closely by a physician to avoid severe negative nitrogen balance and electrolyte changes associated with starvation. Very-low-calorie diets result in significant initial weight loss (15-25% of initial weight) but had high attrition rates (25-50% during the first 3-6 months) and weight regain of 40-50% of lost weight. Long term weight losses were not different between VLCD and low calorie diets. Individuals should be monitored for nutritional adequacy [43, 44]

Carbohydrate

It is recommended to provide 45-65% of total calories from carbohydrate and meet the minimum intake of 130 grams per day [45]. Target total daily fibre of greater than or equal to 14g/1000 kcal per day (DRI). Added sugars should be limited to no more than 25% of total energy [45]. Low glycemic index foods may be incorporated into the diet to assist with glycemic control, increase satiety and reduce hunger. However, a diet with low glycemic index is not recommended specifically for weight management [9].

Low-carbohydrate diets (<35 % of daily calories from carbohydrate) generally are not recommended. Low carbohydrate diets restrict the intake of carbohydrate-containing foods, resulting in a relatively high fat and high protein diet. Individuals should be aware of the following points in regards to low-carbohydrate diets:

- Depletion of glycogen stores results in diuresis and an initial dramatic weight loss.
- Ketones are produced and loss of both adipose tissue and muscle mass occurs during weight loss.
- Compared to reduced calorie diets, some studies have shown more weight loss at 6 months on a reduced carbohydrate diet, but the results were no longer significant at 12 months. They are difficult to sustain over time and maintenance of weight loss is unlikely.
- The diet is low in vegetables and fruit, grain products, and milk and alternatives; therefore, if followed over the long term can increase the risk for nutrient deficiencies and chronic diseases.
- Their safety has not been evaluated for long term use. Caution should be used in suggesting even short term use for individuals with osteoporosis, kidney disease or low LDL cholesterol.

Protein

There is not strong research to guide the estimation of protein requirements for overweight and obese ambulatory individuals. Current recommendations for protein include meeting the DRI-AMDR by providing 10-35% of total daily calories as protein or 1.0 g/kg of ideal body weight (BMI 24.9 kg/m^2). Sufficient intake for most adults is about 60-80 grams per day [9].

Use of adjusted body weight to estimate the metabolically active tissue mass does not improve the accuracy of predicting resting metabolic rate in obese individuals and is not recommended. A common method of using grams/kilogram of actual body weight overestimates protein requirements for obese individuals. For example, using 0.8 – 1.0 g/kg actual weight for 156 kg person, the protein requirement is calculated as 125- 156 g per day. On a 1500 kcal diet, this would represent 33-42% of total calories from protein, exceeding the DRI-AMDR recommendations. Where applicable, assessment of other clinical factors such as renal status, lab values and wound care needs must be considered in the estimation of protein requirements.

Fat

Fat is calorically dense and needs to be limited in order to assist with caloric restriction. It is recommended to limit daily fat to 20-35% of the total daily calories. The amount and type of fat in the diet should follow cardio-protective guidelines [46]. Very-low-fat diets (<15 % total fat) are not recommended for weight management. Caution should be used against the use of such diets because their high carbohydrate content can increase triglyceride levels and their high fibre content (up to 40 to 70 grams daily) can decrease the absorption of calcium, iron and zinc [47].

Fluid Requirements

Guidelines developed for fluid intake for adults are used as fluid requirements for overweight and obese ambulatory individuals are not available. Fluid intake should meet the DRI; adult women 2.7L and men 3.7L per day total water contained in food, beverages and drinking water. Beverage and drinking water intake of 2.2L for women and 3.0L for men should meet these requirements. Intake also needs to be sufficient to satisfy thirst and produce adequate urine output. Fluid intake should not exceed maximum kidney excretion rates (e.g. normal output of 0.7 – 1L/hour)

Assessment of states that increase requirements (e.g. diarrhea, emesis, fever, exercise, medications) and decrease requirements (e.g. cardiac, renal, liver or pulmonary disease) need be included in the estimation of fluid requirements. Common methods of using grams/kilogram of actual or adjusted body weight provide overestimates of fluid requirements for people with obesity. Using 1ml/kcal may underestimate requirements when the total calorie level is restricted (e.g. 1500 mL for 1500 kcal diet).

Table 5. Summary of Nutrition Recommendations for Weight Management and Cardio-protective Guidelines

Energy	
Energy	For weight loss: TEE – (500-1000 kcal) [45]. To maintain body weight and prevent weight gain, balance energy intake and expenditure [42, 48]
Meal Frequency [8]	Three meals plus 1-2 snacks including breakfast. Consumption of greater energy intake during the day may be preferable to evening consumption.
Portion Control [46]	Portion control should be included as part of a comprehensive weight management program. Portion control at meals and snacks results in reduced energy intake and weight loss.
Carbohydrate	
Total	AMDR 45-65% [45] Target midpoint = 55% of total calories. Minimum 130 grams per day [45]. Mostly "complex" carbohydrates- whole grains, fruits and vegetables [42, 45, 49]
Fibre	DRI: 14grams per 1000kcal [45]
Added Sugars	No more than 25% of total energy intake [45]
Sweeteners	Artificial sweeteners can be a part of a calorie reduced diet [8, 50]
Protein	
Total	AMDR 10-35% [45], target 1g/kg IBW or 15-20 % of total calories [4, 48]
Soy	No clear relationship between cooked dry beans and peas and body weight when fed at isocaloric levels [52].
Fat [46]	
Total	AMDR 20-35% [45], target 25 to 35% of total calories [45, 46, 48]
Fat [46]	
Saturated and Trans Fats	<7% saturated and trans fat, with trans fat <1% of total calories [45, 46, 48]
Unsaturated Fats MUFA/PUFA	MUFA 15-20% [45] and PUFA up to 10% of total calories [48]
Omega 3	AMDR 0.6- 1.2% of total calories. Recommend 2 – 4oz servings per week of fish, preferably fatty fish [42]. Cardio-protective targets 500 mg EPA/DHA daily [45, 46]
Nuts	May incorporate 5 oz per week isocalorically into diet, following cardio protective guidelines. Limit or avoid brazil nuts due to higher saturated fat content [51]
Vitamins and Minerals	
Sodium	Target AI = 1500 mg UL =2300mg daily [45]
Calcium	Target DRI 1000-1200 mg daily for adults [45]. and supplement if unable to meet needs with diet alone.
Milk and milk products	Milk and Milk products have no unique role in weight management or body composition [52].
Vitamin D	Provide supplementation as required to achieve normal serum values.
Iron	Meet DRI: 8mg daily for men, 18mg daily for menstruating females [12].
Supplements	A multivitamin is recommended in the following situations: Daily caloric intake of 1500 kcal or less. Less than 6 servings of fruit and vegetables daily. Impaired nutrient absorption Food allergies, dietary restrictions or avoidances. Medication/nutrient interactions.

Fluids	
Fluid	Target the DRI adult women 2.7L and men 3.7L per day total water contained in food, beverages and drinking water [45]. To achieve fluid balance, add 500 mL to total daily urine output.
Alcohol	If consumed, frequency and caloric value needs to be evaluated. Moderate consumption is defined as no more than 1 drink/day for women; no more than 2 drinks/day for men; no more than 5 drinks per week total [53, 54]. Chronic intake of 60g/day (3 or more drinks) associated with increased risk of stroke [46]. Moderate alcohol intake (e.g. one to two drinks per day or 30 grams) can increase HDL-C levels and is associated with a lower prevalence of metabolic syndrome.
Caloric Beverages	Limit intake of calories from beverages as part of a reduced calorie plan High intake (≥25% of daily calories) of beverages with caloric sweeteners is correlated with low HDL levels.
Caffeine	Limit to < 300 mg per day. If > 300 mg per day, recommended to be assessed by a health care provider. If > 600 mg per day, increased risk of anxiety and tachycardia. Maximum dose 1000 mg in 24 hours.
Activity	
Activity	Decrease sedentary/seated/TV/screen time to less than 2 hours per day [1].
Activity	Achieve increase average steps per day. Achieve greater than 150 minutes of moderate intensity activity per week [1, 39].
Behaviour	
Self Monitoring	Record in lifestyle journal for activity, food and beverage intake, thoughts, emotions. Wear a pedometer and record number of steps per day. Use weight scale for weekly body weight measurement. Use kitchen scale and measuring devices to monitor serving sizes of food and beverages. Self monitor health parameters with a glucometer and blood pressure machine.

Meal Replacements

There can be significant variability in the total daily calories consumed due to variety, eating patterns, food availability and portion sizes. People who have difficulty with self selection or portion control may benefit from meal replacements as part of a comprehensive weight management plan. By substituting one or two daily meals or snacks with meal replacements, there is improved consistency of nutrients and calories. There is also improved compliance with hypocaloric diet treatment [55]. Meal replacements can be used a part of a comprehensive strategy for weight loss or weight maintenance. Research shows that there is a greater reduction in weight, even up to 4 years, in people using meal replacements compared to self-selected diets [1, 9].

The meal replacement should provide reduced calories compared to the usual intake at that meal while providing fullness or satiety. Product selection should provide a minimum of 225 calories per serving, are higher in protein, lower in fat and moderate carbohydrate balance [56]. High protein or products developed for diabetes often meet these requirements. Products that are higher in calories (e.g. greater than 1.0 kcal/mL) are generally not recommended for this intervention. For the purpose of weight loss, meal replacements should not be used as a beverage choice in addition to the usual diet. The concern is that people will become over-reliant on products and not learn how to appropriately select foods. More research is required to support the long term use of these products. It is recommended the individual works with a registered dietitian to optimize the nutrition content, palatability and caloric content of their diet.

Health Canada has regulatory requirements for products to be designated as a meal replacement for use with energy restricted diets (**see Table 6**) [56]. Many commercially available products are consumed in a liquid format, available either in a ready-to-drink format or powder that is mixed with water or milk.

There are several products that use various terms similar to "meal replacements" including "formulated liquid diet," "nutritional supplement," "meal replacement for special dietary use," or "pre-packaged meal". These products often do not meet Health Canada's guidelines for nutrient composition of meal replacements for an energy restricted diet [56]. These include some pre-measured, portioned foods such as frozen meals, bars, shakes and powders. Pre-packaged meals, nutritional supplements and foods used as part of a low calorie diet may assist in calorie reduction but cannot be defined as "meal replacements".

Table 6. Nutrient Composition of Meal Replacements for Energy Restricted Diets, Health Canada [56]

Nutrient	Requirements
energy	minimum 225 kcal per serving**
protein	20-35% for product alone; aim for 20% of total energy intake
fat	maximum 35% of energy if sole source of nutrition, maximum 30% of energy
saturated and trans fat	if sole source of nutrition, maximum 15% of energy
linoleic acid	minimum 3% energy
a-linolenic acid (omega 3)	minimum 0.5% energy
ratio N6 :N3	4:1 to 10:1
vitamins and minerals	as listed in column 1, appendix D of reference

** Based on IOM RDA/AI for adult men 19-30 years in 900kcal, and on 4 servings per day (e.g. a serving provides 25% RDA/AI).

Preoperative Liquid Diet

The Preoperative Liquid Diet may be indicated for individuals who require short-term reduction in total calories and carbohydrate to facilitate a reduction in liver volume in preparation for laparoscopic abdominal surgery. The purpose of reducing liver volume prior to laparoscopic surgery is to increase space in the operative field and reduce potential injury to the liver. This intervention is not required for open bariatric surgical procedures unless reduction of liver volume has been specifically identified as an issue. Individuals who are losing weight prior to surgery may achieve the outcomes desired (e.g. reduction of liver volume) and not require or benefit from this intervention. The Preoperative Liquid Diet is for surgical risk reduction and is not indicated as a weight loss intervention.

The Preoperative Liquid Diet reduces energy intake to facilitate weight loss, reduces liver fat content and reduces liver volume [57, 58, 59, 60]. Initial weight loss is, in part, attributed to the reduction of carbohydrate, which has a diuretic effect producing sodium and water loss, ketosis and glycogen depletion [61]. Glycogen reserves are dependant on recent dietary intake, averaging 400 grams in healthy persons. Each gram of stored glycogen binds 3 to 4 grams of water; decreases in liver glycogen may contribute up to 40% of the observed volume reduction [61].

Reductions in weight, visceral and subcutaneous adipose tissue, and liver volume (5.1-18.7%) occurred during the diet intervention (2-12 weeks) [57, 58, 62], The greatest reductions in liver volume occurred in the first two weeks with maximum effect at 8 weeks [57, 58]. Treatment lasting longer than 6 weeks (e.g. up to 12 weeks) produced further reductions in visceral adipose tissue and weight, further significant reductions in liver volume did not occur. Individuals with the most reduction in BMI had the most reduction in liver volume. If significant weight loss occurs (e.g. >3 kg weight loss in 2 weeks), hepatomegaly associated with steatohepatitis will have improved. Attrition increased and individual compliance decreased with longer treatment time due to boredom and fatigue with the diet [57, 58].

Current best practice recommendations include:

- The diet is generally recommended for a minimum of 2 weeks and up to 6 weeks prior to surgery.
- Total energy intake needs to be below total energy requirements in order to facilitate weight loss and mobilize fat from the liver.
- Total carbohydrate intake needs to be restricted to facilitate glycogen loss.
- Total protein and carbohydrate intake needs to be sufficient to protect lean body mass.
- Total fluid intake needs to be sufficient to prevent dehydration.

The Pre-Operative Liquid Diet consists of commercially available liquid nutrition supplements and calorie-free beverages. Referral to a registered dietitian is recommended for nutrition prescription and patient education. Product selection should consider macronutrient composition, medical co-morbidity, availability, cost and palatability for the individual. Higher protein or diabetic meal replacement products are often selected to limit total calories and carbohydrate while providing adequate protein. Products selected should meet Health Canada guidelines for meal replacements as part of an energy-reduced diet or sole source nutrition [56]. Additional calorie-reduced or calorie-free fluids including water are required to meet fluid requirements.

Due to reduced calorie and carbohydrate intake, changes can occur to glycemic levels. Frequent daily blood sugar monitoring is recommended for individuals with diabetes. Blood pressure can also decrease with weight loss and should be monitored. Adjustments to medication may be required.

Nutrition Monitoring and Evaluation

Goals of treatment are determined collaboratively with the patient and the team. Outcomes are defined for each goal, based on the patient and comparative standards. To achieve the goals and outcomes, specific interventions are determined [3].

At each visit, the dietitian monitors the nutrition care indicators to determine if the goals have been achieved or if further intervention is indicated. To monitor progress, the dietitian should:

- Assess understanding and compliance with the nutrition intervention
- Determine if the intervention is being implemented as recommended
- Provide evidence that the intervention is or is not changing the individual's behaviour or status
- Identify positive and negative outcomes
- Gather information indicating reasons for progress or lack of progress
- Support conclusions with evidence

The nutrition care indicators are compared to the reference or comparative standards shown to produce desired outcomes. The most appropriate reference standard or goal needs to be appropriate for the individual's conditions and the individual care setting. Not all individuals are able to achieve a reference standard (e.g. more than 150 minutes of moderate intensity activity per week). A more appropriate goal towards improvement from baseline level of activity can be used to evaluate progress towards this intervention. It is important to evaluate current status in terms of expected outcomes, be able to understand and explain the variance from expected outcomes and help identify factors that help or hinder progress. One must evaluate if continuation of care is indicated. If further intervention will not produce any change or improvement in the indicator, discontinue nutrition care. For weight management, monitoring and evaluation should include the following:

- Activity level
- Adequacy of nutrient intake
- Adequacy of fluid intake, fluid choices (carbonation, calorie intake)
- Blood work (e.g. vitamin and mineral levels, glycemic control, lipid panel)
- Changes in medication or health status
- Eating behaviours (e.g. rate/pace of eating, meal frequency)
- Eating environment
- Gastrointestinal symptoms (e.g. heartburn, emesis, gas/bloating, bowel function, lactose intolerance)
- Hunger, appetite and satiety
- Multivitamin and mineral supplement use and tolerance
- Self monitoring skills

Outcome Indicators [4]

- Selection of foods and fluids consistent with recommendations
- Portion control. Demonstrated understanding of portions of foods and beverages. Understands and applies portion limits to food selections
- Self management of chronic condition(s)
- Ability to use self-monitoring tools
- Demonstrates problem solving skills
- Achieve improvement in nutrition-related chronic conditions
- Achieve and maintain normal serum values (vitamins, glycemic and lipid indices)
- Takes multivitamin and mineral supplements as recommended
- Weight outcomes consistent with guidelines for intervention and time frame
- Use of coping strategies unrelated to food

Nutrition and Bariatric Surgery Education Checklist

The following are education components important to be reviewed with patients prior to surgery in order to have a prepared and informed patient. Refer to Chapter 14 for more information on specific components after surgery.

- Nutrition implications of a bariatric procedure
- Preoperative liquid diet (if required)
- Weight outcomes
- Post surgical diet- full fluid bariatric
- Protein recommendations and supplementation
- Textural progression and transition to solid diet
- Food and beverage recommendations after surgery
- Vitamin and mineral supplement recommendations
- Recommendations for monitoring after surgery (e.g. self monitoring, follow up appointments, bloodwork)
- Signs and symptoms of nutrition-related problems (e.g. food intolerances, dehydration, constipation, nausea, dumping syndrome)

Nutrition Related Behaviours to practice prior to bariatric surgery

- Separation of liquids from solids
- Avoidance of carbonated beverages
- Eating and drinking at a slower rate, practicing mindfulness
- Self monitoring
- Portion/volume limitations

Conclusion

To achieve and maintain health and weight outcomes, significant lifestyle changes are required for a lifetime and include healthy eating habits, regular physical activity, self-monitoring and stress management. Prevention of weight gain is an important clinical outcome and requires ongoing monitoring, nutrition intervention, activity and behaviour modification. Bariatric surgery is an important treatment for obesity. A specialized multidisciplinary team is required to assess, treat, monitor and evaluate the individual, both before and after the surgery. The registered dietitian plays an integral role, working collaboratively with the patient and the interdisciplinary team.

Acknowledgments

The authors wish to acknowledge Nutrition Services, Alberta Health Service for their permission to use the Nutrition Practice Guidelines for Registered Dietitians for Adult

Bariatric Care and the contributions and expertise of the AHS Registered Dietitians and members of the Adult Bariatric Care Nutrition Working Group.

References

[1] Lau DCW, Douketis JD, Morrison KM, Hramiak IM, Sharma AM, Ur E for the Obesity Canada Clinical Practice Guidelines Expert Panel. 2006 Canadian clinical practice guidelines on the management and prevention of obesity in adults and children. CMAJ 2007;176(8):S1-13. Available from: http://www.cmaj.ca/cgi/reprint/176/8/S1.

[2] Canadian Diabetes Association Clinical Practice Guidelines Expert Committee. Clinical practice guidelines for the prevention and management of diabetes in Canada. Can J Diabetes 2008;200;32(suppl 1):S37-S39;[215 pages]. Available from: http://www.diabetes.ca/files/cpg2008/cpg-2008.pdf.

[3] American Dietetic Association. International Dietetics and Nutrition Terminology (IDNT) Reference Manual: Standardized Language for Nutrition Care Process. Second edition. Chicago, Il.2009

[4] Biesemeier CK, Garland J. ADA Pocket Guide to Bariatric Surgery. Weight Management Practice Group. American Dietetic Association. Chicago, Il. 2009

[5] Foster GD, Wadden TA, Vogt RA, Brewer G. What is a reasonable weight loss? Patients'expectations and evaluations of obesity treatment outcomes. *J Consul & Clin Psych* 1997;65(1):79-85

[6] Wamsteker EW, Geenen R, Zelissen MJ, VanFurth EF, Iestra J. Unrealistic weight loss goals among obese patients are associated with age and causal attributions. *J Am Diet Assoc* 2009;109:1903-8.

[7] Linde JA, Jeffery RW, Levy RL, Pronk NP, Boyle RG. Weight loss goals and treatment outcomes among overweight men and women enrolled in a weight loss trial. *Int J Obes* 2005;29:1002-5.

[8] American Dietetic Association. Position of the American Dietetic Association: Weight Management. *J Am Diet Assoc*. 2009;109:330-46.

[9] American Dietetic Association. Adult weight management evidence based guidelines. 2009. Available from: http://www.adaevidencelibrary.com (Membership required).

[10] Health Canada. Nutrient Value of Some Common Foods. 2008. Available from http://hc-sc.gc.ca/fn-an/nutrition/fiche-nutri-data/nutrient_value-valeurs_nutritives-tc-tm-eng.php

[11] Health Canada. Safe use of natural health products. Available from: http://www.hc-sc.gc.ca/hl-vs/iyh-vsv/med/nat-prod-eng.php

[12] American Psychiatric Association. Diagnostic and Statistical Manual of Mental Disorders, 4th Edition-Text Revision(DSM- IV- TR). American Psychiatric Association. Washington, DC. 2000.

[13] Aills L, Blankenship J, Buffington C, Furtado M, Parrott J. ASBMS Allied Health Nutritional Guidelines for the Surgical Weight Loss Patient. *Surgery for Obesity and Related Diseases*. 2008:4;S73-S108

[14] Holick MF. Vitamin D deficiency in obesity and health consequences. *Curr Opin in Endcrinol Diab*. 2006;13:412-418

[15] Mahlay NF, Verka LG, Thomsen K, Merugu S, Salomone M. Vitamin D Status before roux-en-y and efficacy of prophylactic and therapeutic doses of vitamin D in individuals after roux-en-y gastric bypass surgery. *Obes Surg* 2008;19(5):590-4.

[16] Goldner WS, Stoner JA, Thompson J, Taylor K, Larson L, Erickson J, et.al. Prevalence of vitamin D insufficiency and deficiency in morbidly obese individuals: a comparison with non- obese controls. *Obes Surg* 2008;18(2):145-50.

[17] Rucker D, Allan JA, Fick GH, Hanley DA. Vitamin D Insufficiency in a population of health western Canadians. *CMAJ* 2002;166(12):1517-24.

[18] Wortsman J, Matsuoka LY, Chen TC, Lu Z, Holick MF. Decreased bioavailability of vitamin D in obesity. *Am J Clin Nutr* 2000;72(3):690-3

[19] Sanchez-Hernandez J, Ybarra J, Gich I, De Leiva A, Rius Z, Rodriguez-Espinosa J, Peres A. Effects of bariatric surgery on vitamin D status and secondary hyperparathyroidism: a prospective study. *Obes Surg*. 2005; 15(10):1389-95.

[20] Kushner RF. Micronutrient deficiencies and bariatric surgery. . *Curr Opin in Endcrinol Diab*. 2006;13:405-411.

[21] Ernst B, Thurnheer M, Schmid SM, Wilms B, Schultes B. Seasonal variation in the deficiency of 25-hydroxyvitamin D3 in mildly to extremely obese subjects. *Obes Surg* 2009;19:180-83.

[22] Matsuoka LY, Ide L, Wortsman J, MacLaughlin JA, Holick MF. Suscreens suppress cutaneous vitamin D3 synthesis. *J Clin Endocrinol Metab* 1987;64:1165-8

[23] National Institutes of Health, Office of Dietary Supplements. Dietary supplement fact sheet: vitamin D.(Reviewed 24 June 2011). Available from http://ods.od.nih.gov /factsheets/VitaminD_pf.asp.

[24] Institute of Medicine. Otten JJ, Pitzi Hellwig J, Meyers LD-Editors. Institute of Medicine. Dietary Reference Intakes: The Essential Guide to Nutrient Requirements. National Academies Press, Washington DC. 2006.

[25] Health Canada. Multivitamin/Mineral Supplement Monograph- Vitamin D Available from www.healthcanada.gc.ca home/drug and health products/natural health ingredients database.

[26] Cannell JJ, Hollis BW, Zasloff M, Heaney RP. Diagnosis and treatment of vitamin D deficiency. Expert Opinion in Pharmacotherapy. 2008:9(1);1-12

[27] Trang HM, Cole DEC, Rubin LA, Pierratos A, Siu S, Vieth R. Evidence that vitamin D3 increases serum 25-hydroxyvitamin D more efficiently that does vitamin D2. *Am J Clin Nutr* 1998;68:854-8.

[28] Armas LAG, Hollis BW, Heaney RP. Vitamin D2 is much less effective than vitamin D3 in humans. *J Clin Endocrinol Metab* 2004;89(11):5387-91.

[29] Holick MF, Biancuzzo RM, Chen TC, Klein EK, Young A, Bibuld D et al. Vitamin D2 is as effective as vitamin D3 in maintaining circulation concentrations of 25-hydroxyvitamin D. *J Clin Endocrinol Metab*, 2008:93(3);677-81.

[30] Hanley DA, Cranney A, Jones G, Whiting SJ, Leslie WD, Cole DEC et al. Vitamin D in adult health and disease: a review and guideline statement from Osteoporosis Canada. *CMAJ* 2010:182(17)1864-73.

[31] Holick MF. Vitamin D Deficiency. *N Engl J Med* 2007;357:266-81.

[32] Leu JP, Weiner A, Barzel US. Vitamin D Toxicity: Caveat Emptor. *Endocr Pract.* 2008;14(9):1188-1190.

[33] Bjelakovic G, Gluud LL, Nikolova D, Whitfield K, Wetterslev J, Simonetti RG, Bjelakovic M, Gluud C. Vitamin D supplementation for prevention of mortality in adults. Cochrane Database of Systematic Reviews 2011, Issue 7. Art. No.: CD007470. DOI: 10.1002/14651858.CD007470.pub2.

[34] American Dietetic Association. Determination of resting metabolic rate. In: Adult weight management evidence based guidelines. 2006. Available from: http://www.adaevidencelibrary.com (Membership required).

[35] Frankenfield D, Roth-Yousey L, Compher C. Comparison of predictive equations for resting metabolic rate in healthy nonobese and obese adults: a systematic review. *J Am Diet Assoc* 2005;105(5):775-89. Review.

[36] Ireton-Jones C. Adjusted body weight, con: why adjust body weight in energy-expenditure calculations? *Nutr Clin Pract* 2005;20:474-9.

[37] Mifflin MD, St Jeor ST, Hill LA, Scott BJ, Daugherty SA, Koh YO. A new predictive equation for resting energy expenditure in healthy individuals. *Am J Clin Nutr* 1990;51(2):241-7.

[38] Ainsworth BD, Haskell WL, Whitt MC, Irwin ML, Swartz AM, Strath SJ, O'Brien WL, Bassett DR, Schmitz KH, Emplaincourt PO, Jacobs DR, Leon AS. Compendium of Physical Activities: an update of activity codes and MET intensities. *Med & Sci Sport Ex* 2000;S498-515.

[39] *American College of Sports Medicine. Appropriate physical activity intervention strategies for weight loss and prevention of weight regain for adults. Position Stand. Med & Sci Sport Ex 2009;14:459-71. Available from:* www.acsm-msse.org.

[40] Institute of Medicine of the National Academies: Dietary reference intakes for energy, carbohydrate, fibre, fat, fatty acids, cholesterol, protein and amino acids. The National Academies Press. Washington, DC 2002.

[41] Report of the Dietary Guidelines Advisory Committee on the Dietary Guidelines for Americans, 2010. Available from: http://www.cnpp.usda.gov/DGAs2010-DGACReport.htm

[42] Lichtenstein AH, Appel LJ, Brands M, Carnethon M, Daniels S, Franch HA et al. Diet and Lifestyle Recommendations Revision 2006. A Scientific Statement from the American Heart Association Nutrition Committee. *Circulation* 2006;114:82-96.

[43] National Heart, Lung, and Blood Institute in cooperation with the National Institute of Diabetes and Digestive and Kidney Diseases. The clinical guidelines on the identification, evaluation, and treatment of overweight and obesity in Adults: The Evidence Report, NIH Publication No. 98-4083; September 1998. Available from: http://www.nhlbi.nih.gov/guidelines/obesity/e_txtbk/txgd/40.htm.

[44] Tsai AD, Wadden TA. The evolution of Very-Low-calorie Diets: An Update and Meta-analysis. *Obesity* 2006;14(8):1283-93

[45] National Academies of Science. Dietary Reference Intakes for energy, carbohydrate, fibre, fat, fatty acids, cholesterol, protein, and amino acids. National Academies Press, Washington DC. 2005. Available from:http://www.nap.edu/catalog.php? record_id= 10490

[46] American Dietetic Association. Evidence-based guidelines. Disorders of lipid metabolism. 2005 Available from: http://www.adaevidencelibrary.com (ADA membership required).

[47] Strychar, I. Diet in the management of weight loss. *CMAJ.* 2006;174(1).

[48] National Cholesterol Education Program Expert Panel on detection, evaluation, and treatment of high blood cholesterol in adults (Adult Treatment Panel III). Third report of the National Cholesterol Education Program (NCEP) Expert Panel on detection, evaluation, and treatment of high blood cholesterol in adults (Adult Treatment Panel III). *JAMA* 2001;285(19).

[49] Genest J, McPherson R, Frohlich J, Anderson T, Campbell N, Carpentier A et al. 2009 Canadian Cardiovascular Society/Canadian guidelines for the diagnosis and treatment of diyslipidemia and prevention of cardiovascular disease in the adult- 2009 recommendations. *Can J Cardiol* 2009;25(10):567-79.

[50] Welsh J, Sharma A, Abramson J, Caccarion V, Gillespie C, Vos, M. Caloric Sweetener Consumption and dyslipidemia among US adults. JAMA 2010;303(15):1490-1497

[51] Salas-Salvado J, Fernandex-Ballard J, Ros, E, Martinex-Gonzalez MA, Fito M, Estruch R et al. Effect of a Mediterranean Diet supplemented with nuts on Metabolic syndrome status. One year results of the PREDIMED randomized trial. *Arch Int Med* 2008;168(22):2449-58.

[52] Dietary Guidelines for Americans, 2010.Available from http://www.cnpp.usda.gov /DietaryGuidelines.htm

[53] National Institute on Alcohol Abuse and Alcoholism (NIAAA). State of the Science Report on Moderate Drinking 2003.

[54] Dietary Guidelines for Americans (2005) D8: Ethanol. Available from www.health.gov/dietaryguidelines/dga2005

[55] Foster GD, Makris AP, Bailer, BA. Behavioral treatment of obesity. *Am J Clin Nutr* 2005;82(suppl):230S-5S.

[56] Health Canada Appendix D - Proposed Revisions for the Nutrient Composition of Meal Replacements. 2005 Available from http://www.hc-sc.gc.ca/fn-an/nutrition/vitamin /fortification_final_doc_app-ann_d-eng.php#2

[57] Colles SL, Dixon JB, Marks P, Strause BJ, O'Brien PE. Preoperative weight loss with a very-low-energy diet: quantitation of changes in liver and abdominal fat by serial imaging. *Am J Clin Nutr* 2006;84:301-11.

[58] Fris R. Preoperative low energy diet diminishes liver size. *Obes Surg* 2004;14:1165-70.

[59] Lewis MC, Phillips ML, Slavotinek JP, Kow L, Thompson CH, Toouli J. Change in liver size and fat content after treatment with Optifast® very low calorie diet. *Obes Surg* 2006;16:697-701.

[60] Busetto L, Tregnaghi A, DeMarchi F. Liver volume and visceral obesity in women with hepatic steatosis undergoing gastric banding. *Obes Research* 2002;10:408-11

[61] St. Jeor ST, Howard BV, Prewitt E, Bovee V, Bazzarre T, Eckel RH. Dietary protein and weight reduction: a statement for healthcare professionals from the Nutrition Committee of the Council on Nutrition, Physical Activity, and Metabolism of the American Heart Association. Circulation 2001;104:1869-74.

[62] Eid G. Very-low-calorie diet before bariatric surgery reduces risk in superobese patient. American College of Surgeons 94th Annual Clinical Conference. 2008.

In: The Fundamentals of Bariatric Surgery
Editors: Shahzeer Karmali and Daniel W. Birch
ISBN: 978-1-62417-732-3

Chapter 4

Psychiatric Assessment of the Bariatric Patient: Pre-operative

Brian Stonehocker[1] and Margot Steele[2]
[1]Assistant Clinical Professor, University of Alberta, Edmonton, AB, Canada
[2] Weight Wise Bariatric Centre Psychologist, Alberta Health Services, Edmonton, AB, Canada

Abstract

Psychiatric disorders are common in bariatric surgery candidates. Current literature indicates the prevalence of Axis 1 disorders is 20-60%, while personality disorders are reported for 25% of candidates. The role of pre-operative mental health assessment is well established, with most treatment guidelines recommending mental health evaluations be considered for all patients prior to bariatric surgery. Uncontrolled severe psychiatric illness, suicidality, and persistent substance use/dependence are commonly noted as contraindications to bariatric surgery. Related factors such as eating behaviours, compliance, cognition, and emotional functioning can also impact post-operative outcomes.

Although most bariatric surgery programs require some form of mental health intervention, screening varies amongst programs. The role of pre-operative screening is to identify conditions that would increase surgical risk, as well as to identify treatable conditions requiring optimization prior to surgery.

Introduction

The relationship between obesity and psychiatric disorders is complex. Obesity is overrepresented in patients with severe and persistent mental illness such as mood disorders or schizophrenia. These illnesses often present with a symptom profile impacting motivation, energy, and appetite. Moreover, psychotropic medications have metabolic side effects and may contribute to weight gain. Obesity related distress may mimic or exacerbate psychiatric disorders such as depression and anxiety. Amongst patients seeking bariatric surgery, the current prevalence of psychiatric disorders is reported at 20-60%, which is substantially higher than the rates found in the general obese population. The most commonly identified disorders are mood disorders, which have been reported in 10-30% of surgical candidates. Other common disorders include eating disorders (10-40%) personality disorders (25%), and anxiety disorders (10-15%). While current substance use disorders are less common (1-2%), up to 30% of candidates may have a lifetime history of a substance use disorder. The presence of an Axis I or Axis II disorder does not necessarily contraindicate surgery, but may affect the outcome of surgery. The literature is mixed with respect to the impact of psychosocial factors on bariatric surgical outcomes. Some studies have shown similar or even slightly improved surgical outcomes in patients with psychiatric disorders compared to those without mental health concerns. The generalizability of these finding is limited by the fact that most outcome studies have already screened out patients with severe dysfunction. Other studies, however, have found poorer outcomes in those with mental health disorders, particularly those with Binge Eating Disorder. It has been suggested that poorer outcomes are best predicted by severity of symptoms rather than the presence or absence of a disorder. Poor outcomes are not limited to suboptimal weight loss. Higher rates of suicidality have been found in the post-bariatric surgery population, reinforcing the need for appropriate mental health screening and follow up. Identifying candidates who are not yet ready for surgery from a psychiatric perspective can be difficult. This process should include a clinical interview in conjunction with standardized screening instruments for disordered eating and psychiatric illness.

Components of Pre-Surgical Evaluation

The Obesity Society and American Society for Metabolic & Bariatric Surgery Medical guidelines recommend a psychosocial-behavioural evaluation for all patients prior to surgery. In addition, a formal mental health evaluation is recommended for all patients with a known or suspected psychiatric diagnosis. While practice varies amongst surgical sites, the vast majority of programs conduct psychological assessments of patients. Clinical interviews and standardized assessment tools are frequently utilized to identify conditions requiring stabilization prior to bariatric surgery, and to identify patients for whom bariatric surgery may be contraindicated. Psychosocial assessments are typically conducted by a psychologist, psychiatrist, or social worker with experience treating obesity. Ideally the evaluators should be affiliated with the surgical center to facilitate communication with other team members and ensure continuity of care. Evaluators should have experience in clinical diagnosis, and possess an understanding of bariatric surgery and obesity.

Clinical Interview

Many surgical programs conduct standardized screening interviews for surgical candidates. In addition to screening for psychopathology, a clinical interview can be used to assess adherence, cognitive functioning, social supports, degree of self efficacy, and expectations of surgery.

A thorough history should assess for the presence of mood, anxiety, psychotic, and substance use disorders. The impact of symptom profile on current functioning and adherence should be addressed. Information regarding current and past treatments including psychotherapy and medications should also be elicited.

Mood disorders such as Major Depressive Disorder are common among surgical candidates. Atypical depression, a subtype of Major Depressive Disorder, can present with increased need for sleep and food. Psychotropic medications such as antidepressants can also contribute to weight gain.

A thorough risk assessment should identify current self-harm, suicidal ideation or intent. As one of the best predictors of future risk is past behaviour, the evaluation should identify past suicide or self harm attempts, including precipitants and outcomes. Anxiety disorders can often be a barrier to treatment or a trigger for emotional eating.

A history of trauma or childhood sexual abuse has been associated with weight gain. These patients may also experience worsening of mood with weight loss as this can lead to feelings of vulnerability. Attention Deficit Hyperactivity Disorder has been reported for up to 25% of treatment resistant obese patients seeking medical attention. Patients with ADHD often are inattentive to internal cues of hunger and satiety.

Binge eating, skipping meals, and distracted eating are common in this population. In addition to the elements found in a standard clinical interview, emphasis should be placed on eating and dietary styles and previous attempts at weight management.

A history of extreme dieting or food restriction should be of concern. Binge eating and emotional eating are common in surgical candidates. True binges should be differentiated from homeostatic hyperphagia (overeating due to hunger) and hedonic hyperphagia (planned overeating of enjoyed foods). Patients with symptoms of binge eating or significant emotional eating may require psychiatric referral and further treatment.

Standardized Screening and Assessment Tools

Standardized assessment tools are frequently utilized as a component of pre-surgical mental health assessments. Tests should be chosen based on the patient's clinical presentation, and the evaluator should have appropriate training to administer and correctly interpret the results.

The use of self-report measures and standardized testing can potentially uncover concerns not identified in a clinical interview.

These measures can also provide quantitative ratings that can be utilized to measure improvement, or to identify patients requiring additional psychiatric assessment. One should utilize caution in relying solely on self-report scales as candidates may underreport symptoms in hopes of presenting as appropriate for surgery. Additionally, obesity related physical symptoms can falsely elevate depression scores on some scales. While there is no accepted standard for evaluations, commonly utilized measures include:

Beck Depression Inventory – II

This is a 21 item self-administered rating scale, takes approximately 5 minutes to complete, and is one of the most widely utilized instruments for measuring the severity of depression. This inventory is used frequently in the pre-surgical evaluation of bariatric patients.

Beck Anxiety Inventory

A self administered inventory that takes five to ten minutes to complete and can discriminate between anxious and non anxious patients in a clinical population.

Binge Eating Questionnaire (BEQ)

This test consists of 12 demographic questions and 11 multiple choice items specific to eating behaviours. It has been validated in treatment-seeking obese populations, and may be utilized for both diagnosis and screening.

Binge Eating Scale (BES)

The BES is designed to assess binge eating in obese subjects. This 16 item self report scale is useful in detecting binge eating, but does not include the needed criteria to diagnose Binge Eating Disorder.

Minnesota Multiphasic Personality Inventory – 2

This inventory consists of 567 true/false items and is used to assess symptoms of social and personal maladjustment.

Patient Health Questionnaire – 9 (PHQ-9)

The PHQ-9 is a nine item self administered scale that can assess symptoms of depression and identify functional impairment. It identifies which domains of functioning are impacted by depression and provides a severity score.

Structured Clinical Interview for DSM-IV – Axis I (SCID-I)

The SCID-I is a diagnostic exam used to identify Axis I disorders. The interview typically requires 45-90 minutes to complete.

The Three-Factor Eating Questionnaire (TFEQ)

This measure consists of 51 items which measure dietary restraint, disinhibition, and hunger.

The World Health ADHD Self Report Scale (ASRS v.1.1)

This self-report screening scale includes 18 questions about the symptoms of ADHD.

Psychiatric Contraindications to Bariatric Surgery

The role of pre-operative screening is to identify conditions which may have an impact on the outcome or effectiveness of the procedure. Just as the presence of medical comorbidities may add to peri-operative or post operative risk for patients, the presence of psychiatric conditions may lead to adverse or suboptimal outcomes.

A number of papers have reported an increase in suicidality following bariatric surgery. As such, a history of current or recent suicidality is considered to be a contraindication to bariatric surgery. Additionally, patients with active substance abuse or a severe, unmanaged psychiatric disorder should not be routinely offered bariatric surgery.

Caution should be utilized with patients who are unable to understand and appreciate the implications of surgery and behavioural change expected, as well as patients who are non compliant with goal of care and follow up.

Other Psychiatric Considerations

The potential impact of bariatric surgery or weight loss on mental state should be factored into the decision to proceed with surgical intervention. While most patients experience improved mood and quality of life with weight loss, some patients experience a worsening of their mental state. Patients with addictive food behaviours, for example, may replace food with other substances such as alcohol. Binge eating can be exacerbated by excessive caloric restriction. Patients with a history of trauma or abuse can experience increased vulnerability and anxiety with weight loss.

Conclusion

Pre-operative psychiatric assessment of the bariatric patient is important for optimizing surgical outcomes. The goal of this assessment is to identify both psychiatric contraindications to surgery and psychiatric comorbidities of obesity that may be ameliorated to promote post-operative success.

Ideally, pre-operative mental health assessments should include both a clinical interview and standardized assessment tools. A comprehensive assessment can guide pre-operative mental health work up to optimize behavioural, cognitive, and somatic symptoms and minimize post operative risk.

References

Beck AT, Steer RA, Brown GK. BDI-II, Beck Depression Inventory: Manual 2nd ed. Boston: Harcourt Brace and Company, 1996

Butcher, J. N., Dahlstrom, W. G., Graham, J. R., Tellegen, A, & Kaemmer, B. (1989).The Minnesota Multiphasic Personality Inventory-2 (MMPI-2): Manual for administration and scoring. Minneapolis, MN: University of Minnesota Press.

First, MB, Spitzer, R, Gibbon M et.al. Structured Clinical Interview for DSM-IV-TR Axis I Disorders, Research Version, Patient Edition. (SCID-I/P) New York: Biometrics Research, New York State Psychiatric Institute, November 2002.

Gormally J, Black S, Datson S, Rardin D, The assessment of binge eating severity among obese persons. *Addictive Behaviours*, 1982 7(1) 47-55

Greenberg I, Sogg S, M Perna F. Behavioral and psychological care in weight loss surgery: best practice update. *Obesity* (Silver Spring). 2009;17(5):880-4.

Grothe KB, Dubbert PM, O'jile JR. Psychological assessment and management of the weight loss surgery patient. *Am J Med Sci*. 2006;331(4):201-6.

Halmi K, Falk J, Schwartz E. Binge-eating and vomiting: a survey of a college population. *Psychological Medicine* (1981), 11 : pp 697-706

Kalarchian MA, Marcus MD, Levine MD, et al. Psychiatric disorders among bariatric surgery candidates: relationship to obesity and functional health status. *Am J Psychiatry*. 2007;164(2):328-34

Kessler RC, Adler L, Ames M, Demler O, et al. The World Health Organization adult ADHD self-report scale (ASRS): a short screening scale for use in the general population. *Psychological Medicine* (2005), 35 : pp 245-256

Kroenke K, Spitzer RL. The PHQ-9: A new depression and diagnostic severity measure. *Psychiatric Annals* 2002; 32: 509-521.

Mechanick JI, Kushner RF, Sugerman HJ, Gonzalez-Campoy JM, et al. American Association of Clinical Endocrinologists, The Obesity Society, and American Society for Metabolic & Bariatric Surgery Medical guidelines for clinical practice for the perioperative nutritional, metabolic, and nonsurgical support. *Endocr Pract* 2008 Jul-Aug;14 Suppl 1:1-83.

Muhlhans B, Horbach T, de Zwaan M. Psychiatric disorders in bariatric surgery candidates: a review of the literature and results of a German prebariatric surgery sample. *Gen Hosp Psychiatry*. 2009;31(5):414-21.

Munoz DJ, Chen E, Fischer S, et al. Considerations for the use of the Beck Depression Inventory in the assessment of weight-loss surgery seeking patients. *Obes Surg*. 2007;17(8):1097-101.

Rosenberger PH, Henderson KE, Grilo CM. Psychiatric disorder comorbidity and association with eating disorders in bariatric surgery patients: A cross-sectional study using structured interview-based diagnosis. *J Clin Psychiatry*. 2006;67(7):1080-5.

Steer, Robert A.; Beck, Aaron T. Zalaquett, Carlos P. (Ed); Wood, Richard John (Ed), (1997). Evaluating stress: A book of resources., (pp. 23-40). Lanham, MD, US: Scarecrow Education, xvii, 474 pp.

Stunkard A, Messick S. The three-factor eating questionnaire to measure dietary restraint, disinhibition and hunger. *Journal of Psychosomatic Research*. Volume 29, Issue 1, 1985, Pages 71–83.

Taylor V, Stonehocker B, Steele M et. al. An Overview of Treatments for Obesity in a Population With Mental Illness. *Can J Psychiatry*. 2012;57(1):13–20.

In: The Fundamentals of Bariatric Surgery
Editors: Shahzeer Karmali and Daniel W. Birch
ISBN: 978-1-62417-732-3

Chapter 5

Respiratory Assessment of the Bariatric Patient: Pre-operative

Justin C. Sebastian
Royal Alexandra Hospital, Edmonton, Canada

Introduction

This chapter will discuss the preoperative pulmonary evaluation of patients who plan to undergo bariatric surgery.

Morbidly obese patients often have numerous comorbidities that are identified and managed prior to surgery. Although it is possible to study an individual's cardiopulmonary function, it remains difficult to predict how an individual reacts under the stresses of surgery.

There are no uniform standards for the respiratory evaluation of bariatric patients. The intent of this chapter is to suggest an approach prior to surgery. To provide the grounds for this, the chapter will begin by discussing pulmonary physiology in obesity followed by an overview of perioperative complications. Hopefully this provides the rationale for the suggested approach to a respiratory assessment of the bariatric patient.

Discussion

Body mass index (BMI) is commonly used to measure obesity but it does not describe the distribution of fat. A high BMI may not predict the physiological changes on the respiratory system universally. [1] Consequently, a higher BMI may not be more predictive of morbidity. [2]

For descriptive purposes, the physiological changes seen in obesity could be compared to the effects of a "bear hug." Increased weight on the thoracic cage and abdomen can affect chest wall movement, airway size, respiratory muscle function, and lung perfusion. The elasticity or the ability to move the chest wall diminishes with the accumulation of fat. This in turn reduces lung compliance. Furthermore it has been recognized that lung compliance in obese subjects reduces markedly in recumbence when compared to the non-obese. [1] A common and challenging position for postoperative patients.

Reduction in chest wall compliance can lead to heightened demands on the diaphragm. Respiratory muscle endurance can be measured with pulmonary function tests (PFTs) by preforming a maneuver known as maximal voluntary ventilation (MVV). Although this is not routinely measured, respiratory muscle endurance may be reduced by as much as 45% in obese individuals. [3, 4] For an overweight person this endurance can be challenged by upper abdominal surgery, sepsis, metabolic derangement, etc., leading to respiratory failure.

Ventilation and perfusion of the lungs is greatest in the dependent lung zones, which would represent the bases in a seated individual. It is normal for this relationship to change with position but it can also be disrupted by obesity. [1] Overweight individuals tend to have a rapid shallow breathing pattern. Studies have shown that in such people with low functional residual capacity (FRC), a larger percentage of their tidal breathing was distributed to the upper lung zones while lung perfusion remained at the bottom. [5] Airway closure, alveolar collapse, and atelectasis at the lung base are the mechanisms proposed for poor ventilation. This ventilation to perfusion ratio abnormality caused by obesity appears to bear a close relationship to reduction in expiratory reserve volume (ERV). [6]

Obesity can have an affect on pulmonary function. The most commonly encountered abnormity is the reduction in FRC and ERV. ERV describes the volume of air that can be forcefully expired from the end of normal expiration while FRC equals ERV plus reserve volume. In comparison, ERV decreases early on even with modest increase in weight. ERV is further reduced in the supine position as the diaphragm assumes a higher position in the chest. [1] Reductions in FRC and ERV, seen in weight gain, occur exponentially and can be encountered with BMI values < 30 kg/m^2. [7]

Vital capacity and total lung capacity are often maintained unless obesity is extreme. Reduction in these lung volumes, even in over weight individuals, should raise the possibility of intrinsic lung disease. [1]

Usually, in mild obesity, spirometry is normal but simultaneous reduction in forced expiratory volume in 1 second (FEV_1) and forced vital capacity (FVC) can be seen as BMI increases. The FEV_1 to FVC ratio, a measure of airway obstruction, is usually normal unless there is coexistent obstructive airway disease. [1] Reduction in FEV_1 and FVC can be associated with low MVV, indicating the possibility of poor diaphragmatic function. [8]

Changes encountered in PFTs might alert physicians on the potential causes of shortness of breath as the frequency of this complaint seems to be growing in overweight individuals.

Pulmonary Complications Following Bariatric Surgery

Pulmonary complications following weight loss surgery are not uncommon and generally similar to those in the general surgical population. These complications can appear early or late following bariatric surgery.

Some of the commonly encountered respiratory issues include deep vein thrombosis (DVT), pulmonary embolism (PE), pneumonia, respiratory failure, and problems related to obstructive sleep apnea (OSA), chronic obstructive pulmonary disease (COPD), and asthma.

The 30-day mortality following bariatric surgical procedures remains less than 0.1% and is favorable in comparison to other major surgical procedure. [9, 10] Pulmonary embolism (PE) remains a common cause of early mortality and can account for than 50% of deaths. [11] The most common risk factors for fatal PE include prior history of venous thromboembolism (VTE), severe venous stasis disease, poor mobility prior to surgery, BMI > 60 kg/m^2, and obesity hypoventilation. [9, 12] The Michigan Bariatric Surgery Collaborative, one of the largest prospective registries of bariatric surgery patients, demonstrate VTE to be more common following open gastric bypass compared to laparoscopic bypass, gastric band, and sleeve gastrectomy. [9] In addition to standard thromboprophylaxis, it has been shown that extended thromboprophylaxis for 10 days post-discharge with enoxaparin 40 mg subcutaneously once a day reduced the incidence of VTE without increase incidence of bleeding. [13]

Atelectasis is a common precipitant of respiratory failure following weight loss surgery. Although mortality is rare event, it is reported that respiratory failure may account for close to 12% of deaths following weight loss surgery. [14] Standard precautions such as early ambulation and incentive spirometry are most effective. OSA is known factor for postoperative respiratory failure. [15, 16] Prior identification and initiation of continuous positive airway pressure therapy (CPAP) would provide further respiratory optimization.

Obesity is well-established risk factors for developing OSA. While the prevalence of OSA in the general population ranges from 9 to 24%, it is felt to be greater in the general surgical population and as high as 71% in the bariatric surgical patients. [17, 18] Even with adequate healthcare access, up to 80% of OSA has gone undiagnosed. [19, 20].

A recent study found higher prevalence of postoperative complications (44% versus 28%; P value < 0.05) in patients with OSA undergoing non-upper airway surgery compared to controls. Difficulties were mostly attributed to oxygen desaturations. Other complications included higher reintubation rate, prolonged oxygen therapy; cardiac arrhythmias, unplanned ICU transfer, and prolonged hospital stay. [16] In contrast, several other studies have shown no adverse outcomes after withholding CPAP in individuals with known OSA or at high risk of having OSA following weight loss surgery. These studies involved selective surgical procedures, increased observation time and prolonged respiratory monitoring. In addition the authors emphasized the importance of optimizing pulmonary status by aggressive incentive spirometry and early ambulation. [21, 22].

A patient's risk for having sleep apnea can be determined using one of several validated prediction rules or questionnaires such as adjusted neck circumference (ANC) [23] or STOP-Bang (snoring, tiredness, observed apneas, elevated BP, and BMI, age, neck circumference, and male gender) questionnaire. [24] Patients found to be at significant risk of having sleep apnea should undergo a polysomnogram (PSG) to confirm the diagnosis and to determine severity. As waiting periods for PSGs can vary depending on availability, home-based unattended portable testing devices have been suggested, as an inexpensive and readily accessible alternative to an attended in-laboratory PSGs. [25] CPAP is the proven therapy for all severities of OSA. It is considered a safe modality after bariatric surgery without increased risk of anastomotic leaks or increased gastric pouch pressures. [26, 27].

Obesity hypoventilation syndrome (OHS) refers to alveolar hypoventilation in an obese individual, which leads to hypercapnia and is often accompanied by hypoxemia. The incidence of OHS may be as high as 31% in adults with a BMI > 35 kg/m^2 and 48% in individuals with a BMI > 50 kg/m^2. [28, 29] OHS is a distinct entity from OSA. The severity of sleep apnea does not correlate with the presence of OHS and OHS can occur in the absence of OSA. [26] Individuals with OHS experience additional morbidity from complications such as pulmonary hypertension, cor pulmonale, and cardiac failure, polycythemia and pulmonary embolism compared to obese subjects without OHS. [28, 29, 30] A consistent definition for OHS is lacking and various organizations utilize different terminology. Consequently, making a diagnosis of OHS may be difficult. Demonstrating elevation in carboxyhemoglobin on an arterial blood gas (ABG) in the early morning or transcutaneous monitoring during a PSG has been utilized. Each method may have practical implications and limitations. The mainstay of treatment would be noninvasive positive pressure ventilation such as CPAP or bi-level positive airway pressure (BiPAP) therapy.

Shortness of breath is frequently encountered by over weight people. The symptoms may mimic asthma. It has been debated if obesity is linked to asthma or whether symptoms reflect the changes in lung volumes and increased airway resistance. [31, 32] COPD can affect up to one quarter of smokers above the age of 40 and many are unaware or undiagnosed. [33] PFTs are fundamental means of identifying many of these issues.

Pre-operative Pulmonary Assessment of the Bariatric Patient

1) History: Age, gender, and smoking history.
2) Physical examination: Height, weight, neck circumference and BMI. Assessment of oral cavity and determination of Mallampati score. This score is a useful physical finding to predict the ease of intubation and is also a predictor of OSA. [34, 35] Presence of bronchospasm and features of right heart failure should be evaluated.
3) Sleep apnea assessment: The risk of OSA can be determined using validated questionnaires such as ANC or STOP-Bang. Daytime symptoms such as sleepiness can be measured using the Epworth Sleepiness Scale. [36] PSG should be arranged for those who suffer from profound daytime sleepiness or found to be at significant risk for OSA. Attended PSGs (Level I Sleep Study) are the gold standard and is the preferred test in the presence of comorbid conditions such as COPD, heart failure or suspected OHS. Unattended PSGs (Level III Sleep Study) are inexpensive and readily accessible alternative for uncomplicated patients.
4) Pulmonary function testing: Useful to assess respiratory symptoms and to identify obstructive airway diseases or restrictive lung defects.
5) Arterial blood gas: Recommended in individual with BMI > 35 kg/m^2 and critical for those with BMI > 50 kg/m^2 or noted to have significant nocturnal hypoxia or polycythemia.
6) Assessment of thromboembolic disease: Prior history of VTE, venous stasis disease, poor mobility prior to surgery, BMI > 60 kg/m^2, and obesity hypoventilation.

References

[1] Parameswaran K, Todd DC, Soth M. Altered respiratory physiology in obesity. *Can Respir J.* 2006;13:203-10

[2] Yusuf S, Hawken S, Ounpuu S, et al. Obesity and the risk of myocardial infarction in 27,000 participants from 52 countries: A case control Study. *Lancet.* 2005;366:1640-9.

[3] Ray CS, Sue DY, Bray G, Hansen JE, Wasserman K. Effects of obesity on respiratory function. *Am Rev Respir Dis.* 1983;128:501-6.

[4] Koenig SM. Pulmonary complications of obesity. *Am J Med Sci* 2001;321:249-79.

[5] Holley HS, Milic-Emili J, Becklake MR, Bates DV. Regional Distribution of Pulmonary Ventilation and Perfusion in Obesity. *J Clin Invest.* 1967; 46:475-81.

[6] Hurewitz A, Susskind H, Harold WH. Obesity alters regional ventilation in lateral decubitus position. *J Appl Physiol* 1985;59:774-83.

[7] Jones RL, Nzekwu MM. The effects of body mass index on lung volumes. Chest. 2006;130:827-33.

[8] Sahebjami H, Gartside PS. Pulmonary function in obese subjects with normal FEV_1/FVC ratio. *Chest.* 1996;110:1425-9.

[9] Finks JF, Cole KL, Yenumula PR, et al. Predicting risk of serious complications with bariatric surgery: Results from the Michigan Bariatric Surgery Collaborative. *Ann Surg.* 2011;254:633-40.

[10] Dimick JB, Welch HG, Birkmeyer JD. Surgical mortality as an indicator of hospital quality: The problem with small sample size. *JAMA.* 2004;292:847-51.

[11] Melinek J, Livingston E, Cortina G, Fishbein MC. Autopsy findings following gastric bypass surgery for morbid obese. *Arch Pathol Lab Med.* 2002; 126:1091-5.

[12] Sapala JA, Wood MH, Schuhknecht MP, Sapala MA. Fatal pulmonary embolism after bariatric operations for morbid obesity. A 24-year respective analysis. *Obes Surg.* 2003;13:819-25.

[13] Raftopoulos I, Martindale C, Cronin A, Steinberg J. The effect of extended post-discharge chemical thromboprophylaxis on venous thromboembolism rates after bariatric surgery: A prospective comparison trial. *Surg Endosc.* 2008;22:234-91.

[14] Morino M, Toppino M, Forestieri P, et al. Mortality after bariatric surgery: analysis of 13,871 morbidly obese patients from a national registry. *Ann Surg.* 2007;246:1002-7.

[15] Kaw R, Pasupuleti V, Walker E, et al. Postoperative complication in patients with obstructive sleep apnea. *Chest.* 2012;141:436-41.

[16] Liao P, Yegneswaran B, Vairavanathan S, et al. Postoperative complications in patients with obstructive sleep apnea: a retrospective cohort study. *Can J Anaesth.* 2009;56:819-28.

[17] Young T, Palta M, Dempsey J, et al. The occurrence of sleep-disordered breathing among middle-aged adults. *N Engl J Med.* 1993;328:1230-35.

[18] Frey WC, Pilcher J. Obstructive sleep-related breathing disorders in patients evaluated for bariatric surgery. *Obes Surg.* 2003;13:676-83.

[19] Kapur V, Strohl KP, Redline S, et al. Under diagnosis of sleep apnea syndrome in U.S. communities. *Sleep Breath.* 2002;6:49-54.

[20] Young T, Evans L, Finn L, Palta M. Estimation of the clinically diagnosed proportion of sleep apnea syndrome in middle-aged men and women. *Sleep.* 1997;20:705-6.

[21] Jensen C, Tejirian T, Lewis C, et al. Postoperative CPAP and BiPAP use can be safely omitted after laparoscopic Roux-en-Y Gastric Bypass. *Surg Obes Relat Dis*. 2008:4; 512-4
[22] Kurrek MM, Cobourn C, Wojtasik Z, et al. Morbidity in patients with or at high risk for obstructive sleep apnea after ambulatory laparoscopic gastric banding. *Obes Surg*. 2011;21:1494-98.
[23] Flemons WW. Clinical practice. Obstructive sleep apnea. *N Engl J Med*. 2002; 347:498-504.
[24] Chung F, Yegneswaran B, Liao P, et al. STOP questionnaire: a tool to screen patients for obstructive sleep apnea. *Anesthesiology*. 2008;108:812-21.
[25] Skomro RP, Gjevre J, Reid J, et al. *Chest*. 2010;138:257-63.
[26] Huerta S, DeShields S, Schpiner R, et al. Safety and efficacy of postoperative continuous positive airway pressure to prevent pulmonary complication after Roux-en-Y gastric bypass. *J Gastrointest Surg*. 202;6:354.
[27] Weingarten TN, Kindrick ML, Swain JM, et al. Effects of CPAP on gastric pouch pressure after bariatric surgery. *Obes Surg*. 2011;21:1900-5.
[28] Sugerman HJ, Fairman RP, Sood RK, et al. Long-term effects of gastric surgery for treating respiratory insufficiency of Obesity. *Am J Clin Nutr*. 1992;55:597S-601S.
[29] Nowbar S, Burkart KM, Gonzales R, et al. Obesity-associated hypoventilation in hospitalized patients: prevalence, effects, and outcome [comment]. *Am J Med*. 2004;116:1-7.
[30] Kessler R, Chaouat A, Schinkewitch P, et al. The Obesity-hypoventilation syndrome revisited: a prospective study of 34 consecutive cases [comment]. *Chest*. 2001;120:369-76
[31] Ford ES, Mannino DM, Redd SC, et al. Body mass index and asthma incidence among USA adults. *Eur Respir J*. 2004;24:740-44.
[32] King GG, Brown NJ, Diba C, et al. The effects of body weight on airway caliber. *Eur Respir J*. 2005;25:896-901.
[33] Schirnhofer L, Lamprecht B, Vollmer WM, et al. COPD prevalence in Salzburg, Austria: results from the Burden of Obstructive Lung Disease [BOLD] Study. *Chest*. 2007;131:29-36.
[34] Mallampati S, Gatt S, Gugino L, et al. A clinical sign to predict difficult tracheal intubation: a prospective study. *Can Anaesth Soc J*. 1985;32:429-34.
[35] Nuckton TJ, Glidden DV, Browner WS, Claman DM. Physical examination: Mallampati score as an independent predictor of obstructive sleep apnea. *Sleep*. 2006;29:903-8.
[36] Johns MW. Daytime sleepiness, snoring, and obstructive sleep apnea. The Epworth Sleepiness Scale. *Chest*. 1993;103:36-6.

In: The Fundamentals of Bariatric Surgery
Editors: Shahzeer Karmali and Daniel W. Birch
ISBN: 978-1-62417-732-3

Chapter 6

General Medical Preoperative Assessment of the Bariatric Patient: Choosing the Right Patient for Surgery

***Sue D. Pedersen*[1] *and Arya M. Sharma*[2]**
[1] LMC Endocrinology Centre, Calgary, AB, Canada
[2] University of Alberta, Edmonton, AB, Canada

Abstract

The general medical preoperative assessment is a key component of successful bariatric surgery. Before contemplating a surgical approach to weight management, it is essential that the root causes of the patient's obesity have been addressed, explored, and optimized. This includes an assessment for medical and iatrogenic contributors to obesity, and a thorough exploration of psychological contributors and consequences to the weight struggle. It is also essential to assess whether nonsurgical options have been appropriately and adequately explored in the past, and whether the patient is prepared to accept the permanent lifestyle alterations that bariatric surgery will impose upon them.

Several medical conditions have been shown to improve following bariatric surgery, including diabetes mellitus, hypertension, obstructive sleep apnea, dyslipidemia, osteoarthritis, hepatic steatosis, polycystic ovarian syndrome, and urinary incontinence. There is controversy as to whether bariatric surgery is associated with a decrease in mortality; this may vary depending on the patient and their stage of the above disease processes. As such, a system that selects appropriate patients for bariatric surgery based on their functional status and stage of disease may be more appropriate than the currently accepted body mass index criteria.

The medical assessment prior to bariatric surgery should include cardiovascular risk assessment, with consideration for noninvasive stress testing for select patients. Pulmonary testing includes an assessment for possible obstructive sleep apnea, consideration of pulmonary function testing, and planning of perioperative prophylaxis against thromboembolic disease. Diabetes mellitus and hypertension control should be optimized. Evaluation for cholelithiasis, hepatic steatohepatitis, and musculoskeletal health should be undertaken as well.

Introduction

The key to optimizing the success of bariatric surgery is in choosing the appropriate patient for the procedure. First, it is essential that the root causes or contributors to the patient's weight struggles have been identified and dealt with optimally. Next, it must be determined whether every other possible option for weight loss (lifestyle management, +/- medications) have been exhausted, as it is generally preferable to manage weight with lifestyle alteration if at all possible. Finally, in the context of a world where the demand for bariatric surgery far outstrips the supply, caution must be exercised in carefully selecting which patients would benefit most from the procedure. Once the appropriate patient has been selected for surgery, comorbid medical issues and risk stratification must be addressed and optimized prior to undertaking the procedure.

Prior to Contemplating Surgery

Before contemplating a surgical approach to weight management, it is essential that the root causes of the patient's obesity have been addressed, explored, and optimally managed.

Medical and Iatrogenic Causes/Contributors to Obesity

Medical causes of obesity must be addressed and optimized. Hypothyroidism is a common cause of weight gain, which is attributed to the fact that energy expenditure falls proportional to the degree of hypothyroidism. Though unusual to be a cause of dramatic obesity, untreated hypothyroidism can certainly be a contributor and must be ruled out, or managed if present. Despite effective treatment, it is often difficult to shed the excess pounds and return to the baseline body weight.

Cushing's syndrome, which is a condition of excess cortisol production, often results in weight gain, particularly in the abdominal fat distribution. Other features of Cushing's syndrome include type 2 diabetes, hypertension, dyslipidemia, and oligomenorrhea. It can be challenging clinically to distinguish Cushing's syndrome from a patient with visceral obesity and the metabolic syndrome, as many of the clinical features overlap. However, it is crucial to make this distinction clinically, as the treatment of Cushing's syndrome is directed at the cause of the excess cortisol production.

There are several medications which may provide an iatrogenic contribution to obesity, and the use of alternative agents should be considered carefully by the prescribing physician (Leslie *et al* 2007). Medications used in the treatment of diabetes mellitus require careful consideration. Metformin, the first line antihyperglycemic agent, is mildly weight negative. Although several second line agents used to control hyperglycemia cause weight gain (sulfonylureas, thiazolidinediones, insulin), other more recently available agents are weight neutral (DPP-IV inhibitors), or can cause substantial weight loss (GLP-1 agonists) (Table 1). In the bariatric population, many patients are severely insulin resistant, necessitating high doses of insulin therapy. Appropriate optimization of the glycemic medication strategy, and response both in terms of glycemic control and weight, must be ensured prior to contemplation of bariatric surgery as a management strategy.

In the realm of antidepressive agents, tricyclic antidepressants are associated with significant weight gain, whereas some selective serotonin reuptake inhibitors have been associated with weight loss. The antiepileptic drugs valproate and carbemazepine are associated with weight gain, whereas the antiepileptic drug topiramate is currently under study in combination with an amphetamine, phentermine, as a potential combination weight loss agent. Extreme care must be exercised in consideration of altering antidepressive medications, in that decompensation of a known psychological illness may precipitate weight gain, as well as threaten the success of bariatric surgery. Glucocorticoids, which are used to treat a wide array of conditions, cause weight gain and a Cushing's phenotype.

Table 1. Commonly Prescribed Medications Affecting Weight*

Category	Drugs that cause Weight Gain	Possible Alternatives
Diabetic medications	Insulin Sulfonylureas Thiazolidinediones	Metformin GLP-1 agonists DPP-IV inhibitors Alpha glucosidase inhibitors
Antidepressants	Amitriptyline Nortryiptyline Clomipramine Imipramine Doxipen Paroxetine Mirtazapine	Other SSRIs Buproprion
Anticonvulsants	Valproate Carbemazapine Gabapentin	Topiramate Lamotrigine
Antipsychotics	Olanzapine Clozapine Quetiapine Respiridone	Haloperidol Aripiprazole

*This table is not an exhaustive list; commonly prescribed medications are represented where alternatives exist.

Psychological Issues

From a psychological perspective, there are many issues that can arise, both as a cause and/or a consequence of the patient's weight struggles; chapter 4 explores these crucial issues in detail. If the patient's psychological relationship with food is not adequately addressed prior to surgery, this can have disastrous postoperative consequences. For example, a patient with binge eating disorder who has not had the disease adequately managed is at risk of binging events postoperatively, which could result in intestinal perforation in a worst case scenario. Substance abuse tendencies must also be addressed and managed, as patients who display addictive tendencies may be more likely to engage in substance abusive behaviors postoperatively.

Have Nonsurgical Options Been Adequately Explored?

It is also essential that nonsurgical options to manage the patient's obesity have been extensively explored with the patient over time. Has the patient been appropriately counseled regarding appropriate permanent lifestyle changes? Has the patient kept a food log over the long term? Does the patient wear a pedometer, and is he or she cognizant of attempting to get enough activity? Bariatric surgery must never be viewed as a quick fix or a first option in the management of obesity; rather, it must be clear to the patient that surgery results in dramatic lifestyle alteration, and should only be considered in the event that other options to manage the patient's weight struggles has proven ineffective for that individual.

Realistic Expectations

Finally, in the discussion of bariatric surgery, it is important to understand the patient's expectations regarding weight loss, and whether those expectations are realistic. A normal range body weight is likely unobtainable for many in this population. It must be understood by the patient that the benefits to weight loss go far beyond the cosmetic, and that the impact on comorbidities of obesity are likely to be substantial. These issues are discussed further in Chapter 4.

What Medical Conditions are Likely to Benefit from Bariatric Surgery?

Many medical conditions associated with obesity have been shown to improve with bariatric surgery.

Diabetes Mellitus

Perhaps one of the most fascinating changes seen after bariatric surgery is the improvement in type 2 diabetes mellitus that is very frequently observed. In the Swedish Obese Subjects trial, which was a prospective, controlled trial of patients undergoing a variety of bariatric surgical procedures, the remission rate of T2DM was found to be 72% at 2 years, compared to 21% in the control group. Studies examining remission rates of T2DM by procedure have found the remission rate to vary from the range of about 55% with gastric banding, 47-66% with sleeve gastrectomy (Lee *et al* 2011, Gill *et al* 2010) , 80-85% with Roux en y gastric bypass, to as high as 95% with biliopancreatic diversion. While these remission rates appear to be sustained at 2 years, longer term studies suggest that about half of these diabetes cases recur by 5 years postoperatively.

The mechanisms of diabetes remission are multifactorial. Decreased caloric intake is one mechanism that is involved with all of the procedures. With weight loss, insulin resistance is decreased, and diabetes improves in line with the decrease in insulin resistance seen.

With gastric bypass surgery, an increase in incretin release is seen from the first introduction of oral food after surgery; this is thought to be due to the presentation of freshly digested nutrients much further down the small intestine.

Sleeve gastrectomy also demonstrates a marked improvement in diabetes well before weight loss. The faster delivery of nutrients to the small intestine is thought to stimulate an increased incretin response as well, which is likely to be a major mediator of the improvements seen.

Factors associated with an increased likelihood of remission of T2DM include a shorter duration of T2DM and lower preoperative glycemic medication requirements.

Cardiovascular Disorders and Other CV Risk Factors

Hypertension has been noted to resolve in 62% of patients and improve in 79% of patients undergoing bariatric surgery, with better results seen with RYGB as compared to gastric banding. Dyslipidemia improves in 70% as well. Atherosclerotic disease has been shown to improve following bariatric surgery, due to reduction in these vascular risk factors, as well as other mechanisms including a decrease in serum inflammatory markers, improvements in endothelial function, and beneficial alterations in coagulation factors. However, the durability of these changes over time remains unclear.

Cardiac function improves postoperatively, with benefits seen including a decrease in left ventricular mass and hypertrophy, improvements in right ventricular function, and improved cardiac performance overall.

Other Comorbidities

Respiratory complications of obesity often improve following bariatric surgery. Obstructive sleep apnea resolves in over 80% of patients in some series, with the frequency of respiratory events (eg apneas and hypopneas) improving for most patients. Restrictive lung disease improves with reduction in body weight as well. These issues are considered in further detail in Chapter 5.

Osteoarthritis symptoms in weight bearing joints improve for most patients following surgery, particularly at the hip, knee, and ankle. Improvements are seen within the first six months to one year postoperatively, with the greatest improvements seen in those with less severe cartilaginous damage at baseline. Weight loss facilitated by bariatric surgery can also enable joint replacement surgery in patients who were previously considered to be at excess operative risk due to their weight.

Gastroesophageal reflux disease (GERD) can improve following bariatric surgery, though this varies with the procedure chosen, as the shape of the stomach can influence the risk of GERD. Sleeve gastrectomy may increase risk of GERD, while RYGB appears to decrease GERD. Hepatic steatosis, which can lead to fibrosis and cirrhosis, improves with bariatric surgery-induced weight loss.

In terms of genitourinary disease, polycystic ovarian syndrome almost invariably improves with bariatric surgery-induced weight loss. Urinary incontinence symptoms often improve or resolve completely (Kaul & Sharma, 2011).

Effect on Mortality

The effect of bariatric surgery on mortality is controversial. Two landmark studies in populations that were primarily female patients demonstrated a decrease in mortality with mixed procedures and with gastric bypass surgery (Sjöström *et al* 2007, Adams *et al* 2007). A more recent analysis of the SOS study shows a small but significant reduction in cardiovascular mortality. A retrospective study of predominantly older male patients did not show a mortality benefit (Maciejewski *et al* 2011). It is plausible that the effect of bariatric surgery to decrease mortality may vary depending on the patient and their stage of the above disease processes.

Choosing the Right Patient for Bariatric Surgery: Who is Most Likely to Benefit?

In a world where the number of patients who may be candidates for bariatric surgery far outstrips the limited supply, a high degree of selectivity must necessarily be applied in choosing which patients may benefit most from these procedures. The NIH has established criteria based on BMI; namely, a patient with BMI ≥40, or ≥35 with at least one serious comorbidity (type 2 diabetes, obstructive sleep apnea, obesity related cardiomyopathy, or severe osteoarthritis) would qualify. As the remission rates of T2DM are so impressive, many groups of bariatric physicians worldwide have proposed that the BMI criteria be lowered to ≥30 in the case of a patient with T2DM. However, use of BMI criteria alone is subject to significant limitation, as a BMI cutoff does not take into account the degree of medical complications that a patient has, and therefore is not an appropriate indicator (taken alone) of who may benefit most from these surgeries. For example, a patient with a BMI of 42 with T2DM and hypertension may stand to benefit from bariatric surgery more than a patient with the same BMI but without any complications. In addition, from a cost efficacy perspective, the cost savings in terms of QALY over the long term is much higher for a patient in whom complications of obesity have been improved or resolved, compared to a patient that is free of complications of obesity. An alternative method of assessment of the status of a patient with obesity is the Edmonton Obesity Staging System. This system can be applied to any patient with a BMI ≥25; classifications are as follows:

EOSS STAGE	DESCRIPTION
0	No apparent risk factors (e.g., blood pressure, serum lipid and fasting glucose levels within normal range), physical symptoms, psychopathology, functional limitations and/or impairment of well-being related to obesity
1	Presence of obesity-related subclinical risk factors (e.g., borderline hypertension, impaired fasting glucose levels, elevated levels of liver enzymes), mild physical symptoms (e.g. dyspnea on moderate exertion, occasional aches and pains, fatigue), mild psychopathology, mild functional limitations and/or mild impairment of well-being
2	Presence of established obesity-related chronic disease (e.g., hypertension, type 2 diabetes, sleep apnea, osteoarthritis), moderate limitations in activities of daily living and/or well-being
3	Established end-organ damage such as myocardial infarction, heart failure, stroke, significant psychopathology, significant functional limitations and/or impairment of well-being
4	Severe (potentially end-stage) disabilities from obesity-related chronic diseases, severe disabling psychopathology, severe functional limitations and/or severe impairment of well-being

The EOSS thus provides a pragmatic staging tool, which goes far beyond BMI, to take into consideration the impact of excess adipose tissue on the disease status of the patient. The EOSS has been shown to be predictive of mortality risk, with scores of 2 and 3 being associated with increased mortality risk compared with scores of 0 or 1, even after adjustment for BMI and the metabolic syndrome (Padwal *et al* 2011). It has been suggested that the EOSS staging system be utilized to prioritize patients for bariatric surgery, with patients of EOSS stage 2-3 being the most appropriate surgical candidates.

Preparing the Patient for Surgery

This section reviews the medical aspects of preoperative preparation; nutritional and psychological preparation are discussed in chapters 3 and 4, respectively.

Cardiac Risk Assessment

Cardiovascular risk assessment must be considered before proceeding with surgery of any kind. As the bariatric patient has an increased risk of cardiovascular disease, heart failure, sleep apnea with or without pulmonary hypertension, and pulmonary embolic disease, the importance of cardiovascular risk stratification is an integral component of preoperative evaluation.

The initial cardiovascular evaluation begins with the history, physical examination, and an electrocardiogram (EKG). Important historical variables to enquire about include:

- any past history of atherosclerotic disease
- symptoms of cardiac ischemia
- symptoms of congestive heart failure (exertional dyspnea, orthopnea, paroxysmal nocturnal dyspnea)
- symptoms of peripheral vascular disease (eg intermittent claudication)
- any past history of venous or arterial thrombosis

Functional status is important to assess, as a good functional capacity is associated with a lower risk of complications. Appropriate questions to ask are whether a patient is able to ascend one flight of stairs or walk 4 blocks on a level plane. These activities correspond to approximately 4 METs (metabolic equivalents); ability to perform 4 METs or better is associated with a lower risk of general anesthesia. In the bariatric population, dyspnea and decreased functional capacity may be present due to the obesity itself rather than cardiovascular disease, which makes the assessment more uncertain in this population.

The physical exam must include BP measurement with an appropriately sized cuff, complete cardiopulmonary exam, and examination of the extremities for edema and peripheral vascular disease. Peripheral edema may be due to decreased lymphatic drainage in this population, but an echocardiogram must be conducted in any patient with this finding.

Should a patient have any major predictors of high cardiac risk based on the above assessment (eg unstable angina, NYHA Class IV congestive heart failure, significant arrhythmia), surgery should be delayed until the issue in question is managed appropriately; in some cases, the cardiologist or internist involved may recommend against bariatric surgery altogether due to excess operative risk.

Table 2. Lee Score For Assessment of Perioperative Cardiovascular Risk

Six independent predictors of major cardiac complications
High-risk type of surgery (examples include vascular surgery and any open intraperitoneal or intrathoracic procedures)
History of ischemic heart disease (history of MI or a positive exercise test, current complaint of chest pain considered to be secondary to myocardial ischemia, use of nitrate therapy, or ECG with pathological Q waves; do not count prior coronary revascularization procedure unless one of the other criteria for ischemic heart disease is present)
History of Heart Failure
History of cerebrovascular disease
Diabetes mellitus requiring treatment with insulin
Preoperative serum creatinine >177 µmol/L
Estimated % risk of perioperative cardiovascular event, based on number of above predictors
No risk factors (Lee Score = 0): 0.5%
One risk factor (Lee Score = 1): 1%
Two risk factors (Lee Score = 2): 4-7%
Three or more risk factors (Lee Score $\geq$ 3): 9-11%

If the patient does not have any major predictors, risk can then be stratified using a risk model such as the Lee Score (Table 2). To calculate the Lee Score (Lee *et al* 1999), one point is assigned for each of six variables, which each represent predictors of major cardiac complications. This score then corresponds to an estimated risk of perioperative cardiac event. In patients with a Lee Score of 2 or greater, consideration should be given for noninvasive cardiovascular stress testing, particularly if functional capacity is low. That being said, stress testing is often difficult in this patient population, as functional capacity may limit the ability to perform exercise stress testing, and body size and/or morphology may limit the ability to perform dobutamine echocardiogram or dipyridamole thallium scintigraphy.

Prevention of venous thromboembolic disease in the perioperative period must also be planned, as both obesity and general surgery are risk factors. Unfractionated or low molecular weight heparin should be utilized perioperatively, and continued until the patient is fully mobilized. Most centers additionally utilize mechanical prophylaxis in the form of intermittent pneumatic compression stockings applied to the lower extremities while the patient is bedridden, though caution must be taken that the application of these devices does not inadvertently inhibit mobilization postoperatively.

Pulmonary Assessment

A thorough pulmonary assessment is part of the routine preoperative evaluation of the bariatric patient, as these patients are at risk of both obstructive and restrictive lung disease (see Chapter 5). Risk factors for pulmonary operative complications include older age, chronic obstructive lung disease, obstructive sleep apnea, congestive heart failure, and lower overall functional capacity.

The assessment begins with the history, physical examination, and functional capacity, including assessment regarding the above risk factors. Smoking cessation should occur at least 8 weeks prior to surgery. A chest x-ray is done routinely, though the yield for patients without any pulmonary signs or symptoms is small. If a patient is suspected of having obesity hypoventilation syndrome, arterial blood gases (ABG) should be measured. Pulmonary function testing is conducted in most patients as well.

Obstructive sleep apnea may be present in as many as 50% of patients presenting for bariatric surgery; preoperative evaluation for this condition is paramount (see Chapter 5). Diagnostic polysomnography should be considered; nasal CPAP is recommended in most cases where OSA is diagnosed. OSA is also associated with airway characteristics that may pose difficulties in perioperative airway management.

Diabetes Management

Glycemic control should be optimized prior to bariatric surgery. Elevated blood glucose perioperatively for any surgical procedure increases the risk of infection and other operative complications. For some patients having bariatric surgery, preoperative control may prove difficult – 'refractory' or poorly controlled diabetes may in fact have been an important criterion in the selection of the patient for surgery in the first place. Patients with severe obesity can be extremely insulin resistant, which can necessitate high doses of insulin to get glycemic control. However, it should be emphasized that in most cases, insulin can be titrated to effectively reach blood glucose targets.

Immediately postoperatively, due to the dramatic decrease in caloric intake, as well as to alteration in incretin hormones (in the case of gastric bypass and sleeve gastrectomy in particular), a dramatic improvement in glycemia is often seen. This can necessitate a dramatic decrease or complete cessation in need for insulin or oral hypoglycemic agents. The reader is referred to Section 4 for further discussion on postoperative management.

Hypertension

As adipose tissue plays an important role in the pathogenesis of hypertension (see Chapter 2), hypertension is a condition that affects a significant proportion of bariatric patients. These patients often require several medications for control. Prior to surgery, blood pressure should be well controlled, defined as BP $\leq$ 140/90, or $\leq$ 130/80 in diabetics.

Gastrointestinal

The presence of cholelithiasis in the bariatric population is a very common comorbidity. This association is likely multifactorial, including morbid obesity, past history of rapid weight loss, and the prevalence of female gender in this population. Following gastric bypass surgery, the incidence of stone or sludge formation has been shown to exceed 30%, though this risk can be substantially decreased with the use of ursodeoxycholic acid (Shiffman *et al* 1991).

Should a patient develop ascending cholangitis of the common bile duct due to an obstructing stone following gastric bypass surgery, management can be challenging, as it is technically very difficult to access the ampulla (entrance to the common bile duct) to release the stone endoscopically due to the anatomic alterations of gastric bypass surgery.

Preoperative evaluation of the bariatric patient can include abdominal ultrasound, both for visualization of hepatic anatomy as well as presence of gallstones. It remains controversial as to whether cholecystectomy should be performed simultaneously with gastric bypass surgery if gallstones are present. Chapter 7 will discuss the role of endoscopy and H.pylori screening in bariatric patients.

Non alcoholic fatty liver disease (NAFLD) is common in this population, and is discussed in detail in chapter 2. Liver enzymes should be checked preoperatively; further evaluation should be considered if levels are increased 2-3 times upper limit of normal or more.

Musculoskeletal

Patients with obesity are at increased risk of gout. Surgical procedures are risk factors for gout attacks, as is rapid weight loss of any cause. For patients with frequent attacks of gout, prophylactic therapy can be considered (Mechanick *et al*, 2008).

Although obesity tends to be associated with increased bone mass, low vitamin D and secondary hyperparathyroidism are often seen. Further, there is evidence to suggest an increased risk of osteoporosis years following malabsorptive bariatric procedures such as RYGB. Preoperative biochemical screening with serum 25 vitamin D, PTH, and markers of bone metabolism should be considered, and bone density testing may be helpful in select patients who are at risk of metabolic bone disease.

References

Adams TD, Gress RE, Smith SC, et al. Long-term mortality after gastric bypass surgery. *N Engl J Med* 2007; 357:753.

Gill RS, Birch DW, Shi X, Sharma AM, Karmali S. Sleeve gastrectomy and type 2 diabetes mellitus: a systematic review. *Surg Obes Relat Dis*. 2010;6(6):707-13.

Kaul, A and Sharma, J. Impact of bariatric surgery on comorbidities. *Surg Clin N Am.* 2011;91(6):1295-1312.

Lee TH, Marcantonio ER, Mangione CM, Thomas EJ, Polanczyk CA, Cook EF, Sugarbaker DJ, Donaldson MC, Poss R, Ho KK, Ludwig LE, Pedan A, Goldman L. Derivation and prospective validation of a simple index for prediction of cardiac risk of major noncardiac surgery. *Circulation*. 1999;100(10):1043-9.

Lee WJ, Chong K, Ser KH, Lee YC, Chen SC, Chen JC, Tsai MH, Chuang LM. Gastric bypass vs sleeve gastrectomy for type 2 diabetes mellitus: a randomized controlled trial. *Arch Surg*. 2011;146(2):143-8.

Leslie WS, Hankey CR, Lean ME. Weight gain as an adverse effect of some commonly prescribed drugs: a systsematic review. *QJM* 2007;100:395.

Maciejewski ML, Livingston EH, Smith VA, et al. Survival among high-risk patients after bariatric surgery. *JAMA* 2011; 305:2419.

Mechanick JI, Kushner RF, Sugerman HJ, Gonzalez-Campoy JM, Collazo-Clavell ML, Guven S, Spitz AF, Apovian CM, Livingston EH, Brolin R, Sarwer DB, Anderson WA, Dixon J. American Association of Clinical Endocrinologists, The Obesity Society, and American Society for Metabolic and Bariatric Surgery medla guidelines for clinical practice for the perioperative nutritional, metabolic, and nonsurgical support of the bariatric patient. *Surg Obes Relat Dis*. 2008;4(5 Suppl):S109-84.

Padwal RS, Pajewski NM, Allison DB, Sharma AM. Using the Edmonton obesity staging system to predict mortality in a population-representative cohort of people with overweight and obesity. *CMAJ.* 2011;183(14):E1059-66.

Shiffman ML, Sugerman HJ, Kellum JM, Brewer WH, Moore EW. Gallstone formation after rapid weight loss: a prospective study in patients undergoing gastric bypass surgery for treatment of morbid obesity. *Am J Gastroenterol*. 1991;86(8):1000-5.

Sjöström L, Narbro K, Sjöström CD, et al. Effects of bariatric surgery on mortality in Swedish obese subjects. *N Engl J Med* 2007; 357:741.

Section 3: Operative Management of Bariatric Patient-Procedure, Mechanisms of Action, Outcomes

In: The Fundamentals of Bariatric Surgery
Editors: Shahzeer Karmali and Daniel W. Birch
ISBN: 978-1-62417-732-3

Chapter 7

The Laparoscopic Adjustable Gastric Band: *Key Concepts*

Daniel W. Birch
University of Alberta, Edmonton,
Alberta, Canada

Abstract

The laparoscopic adjustable gastric band (LAGB) is an important procedural option in the surgical management of severe obesity. In this chapter, key concepts and principles will be introduced for the LAGB. Included in this review will be a discussion on the mechanism of action, patient preparation and selection, an operative overview and details on post-operative management and clinical outcomes.

This should enable the reader to have an appropriate discussion with patients and health care providers on key features of the LAGB.

Introduction

The laparoscopic adjustable gastric band (LAGB, Figure 1) remains the least complex, evidence-based surgical treatment option for sustainable weight loss in patients with severe obesity.

With over 15 years of scientific study and evidence in support of its clinical safety and weight loss sustainability, this simple and effective surgical intervention is an important treatment option for patients and bariatric surgeons. In this chapter, fundamental principles of the LAGB will be reviewed to facilitate trainees, physicians and health care professionals' understanding of the LAGB and to begin to manage patients with this surgical device accordingly.

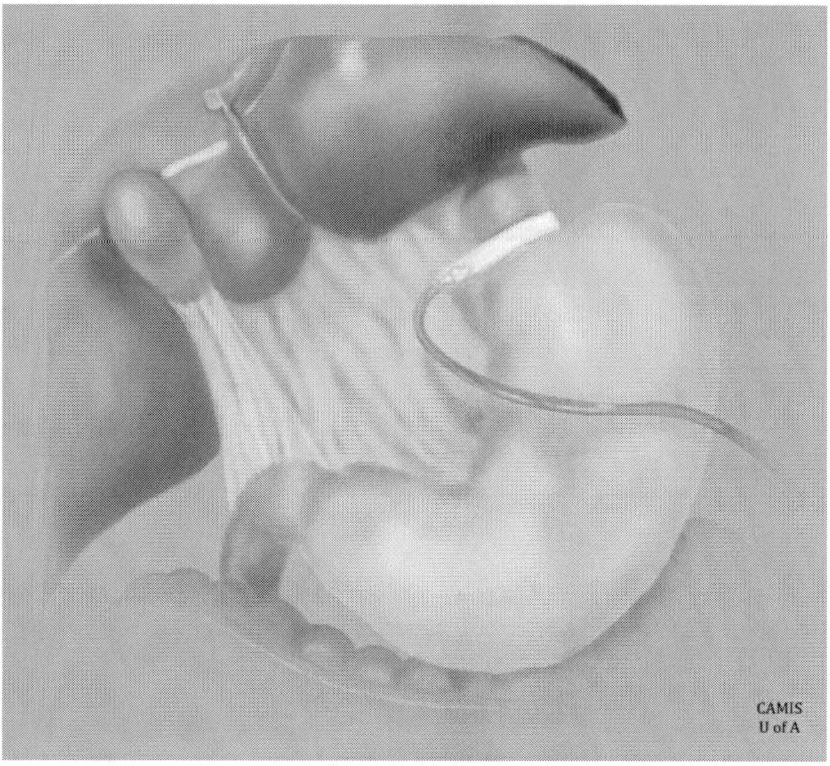

Figure 1. CAMIS LAGB.

Brief History of the LAGB

The initial interventions using gastric banding for weight loss involved non-adjustable, synthetic gastric bands placed by laparotomy. Wilkinson is credited with the initial reported procedure in 1978 and subsequently published outcomes with this procedure. Materials used for early bands included polypropylene and goretex. Mesh erosion and frequent vomiting were among the complications that plagued this initial technique. Kuzmak subsequently developed an adjustable gastric band and is believed to have placed the first device by open surgery in 1986. Cadiere reported the first laparoscopic adjustable band placement in 1992.

Currently, there are a number of LAGBs produced by different manufacturers around the world, however the most common bands are the Swedish adjustable gastric band (Realize band, Johnson and Johnson/Ethicon Endosurgery) and the Lap-Band (Allergan).

Mechanism of Action

Gastric bands partition the stomach and create a very small gastric pouch. With appropriate nutritional strategies by the patient, the small pouch limits meal portion size by creating early satiety. When the gastric band is appropriately filled, the small pouch empties slowly and the satiety is prolonged.

Adjusting the LAGB is based on feedback from the patient following inquiries by dieticians, physicians and surgeons on meal tolerance, extent of satiety and presence of 'negative' or untoward clinical signs such as nausea and vomiting.

There are several critical features and limitations of the LAGB that must be learned (by physicians and patients!) and implemented in bariatric clinics to achieve satisfactory clinical outcomes:

'Pearls' of the LAGB:

1) Selection: selecting or 'matching' patients to the LAGB is paramount to success (vs other surgical options)
2) Acceptance: the characteristics of LAGB-induced weight loss (based on evidence) must be acceptable to the patient i.e. a slow and steady weight loss (over 1-2years) is typical to an average of 50-60 pounds
3) Restriction: creating restriction through LAGB adjustment should be a gradual process and will not drive lifestyle change, it *reinforces* this change and facilitates long term compliance
4) Follow-up: beware the vomiting patient – this is always an indication of nutritional/lifestyle struggles or band complications (imaging of band position may be necessary).

The Bariatric Clinic Process in Preparation for LAGB

There are critical aspects to the bariatric clinic that are covered elsewhere in this book, however several key principles of the pre-operative process should be reiterated here for effect.

Obesity is a complex, chronic disease, therefore a thorough assessment of each patient will be required pre-operatively and an appropriate team of health care consultants will be necessary to complete this process, including: physician/bariatricians, dieticians, nursing, mental health professionals and surgeons (the team is not limited to this list, and all members of the team must be properly trained or experienced in obesity medicine and bariatric surgery – 'run of the mill' health care professionals with little or no experience in obesity medicine are inappropriate in this clinical setting).

The team should contribute to a thorough assessment for each patient, confirming they have 'readiness' for lifestyle change, stable and supportive social and family circumstances, treated mental illness with a focus on adult attention deficit disorder, awareness and preparation for the need for change in both nutritional and physical aspects of their lives (specific nutritional plans may be helpful) and an adequate understanding of the need for access to and follow-up in a structured multidisciplinary bariatric clinic.

Patient Selection

Once the patient is considered an appropriate candidate for bariatric surgery, a discussion should take place presenting several options for bariatric surgery. In this discussion, the procedures can be contrasted and compared in terms of overall complexity, technical features, peri-operative risk and long term complications, expected clinical outcomes (ie weight loss), limitations, reversibility and impact on long term health and treatment (see Figure 2 for a guide to discussion with patients).

The LAGB may be the most appropriate option for a patient who: desires the least complex, safest option for bariatric surgery (peri-operative risk), requires 50-60 pounds of weight loss, accepts the concept of a 'foreign body', desires/needs reversibility as a feature (future pregnancy is desired in women), and is accepting of the post-operative process that will slowly adjust the restriction of the band to reinforce and support their lifestyle change.

	Band	Sleeve	Gastric Bypass
Safety			
Reversibility			
Complexity			
Nutritional impact			
Foreign Body			
Restricted Meds			
Long term data			
Weight loss	(50 lb)	(70 lb)	(80 lb)

Figure 2. Decision aid.

Procedure Planning

Although experts differ, the presence of a hiatus hernia may complicate placement of the LAGB. It is reasonable therefore, to consider imaging of the esophagus and stomach pre-operatively thorough fluoroscopic assessment using barium or esophagogastroscopy. A large hiatal hernia with a distinct sac should be considered a relative contraindication to placement, and patients should be considered for other surgical options. The rationale for this approach is related to the relatively poor long term outcomes of primary hiatal hernia repair (specifically recurrence rates), and the accompanying disruption of the posterior anatomic space that should be preserved to maintain LAGB position.

Pre-operative weight loss should only be necessary in those patients who are considered at risk for clinically significant hepatomegaly (creating problems with liver retraction and visibility of the proximal stomach) and visceromegaly (creating challenges with gastroepiploic fat retraction).

There is evidence to support pre-operative weight loss in this sub-population of severely obese patients, however it is not clear how to select this group. Determining which patients have severe hepatomegaly may be facilitated through clinical suspicion (male gender, central distribution of excess body weight) or imaging (CT based volumetric assessment of anatomic left lobe of liver).

Pre-operative weight loss may be achieved through lifestyle change or calorie reduction with meal replacement strategies (typically balanced liquid nutritional substitutes). In clinical scenarios of greatest concern or risk, loss of 10% of baseline weight may be necessary to resolve severe hepatomegaly or visceromegaly.

Liquid nutritional substitutes given pre-operatively may compromise post-operative patient outcomes. It is not uncommon in the post-operative period to identify patients who surreptitiously resort to these liquid substitutes (sweet and satisfying!) and inadvertently sabotage their own clinical success. This may be most important in patients with the LAGB who are trying to refrain from consuming liquids with meals (to get the greatest degree of meal-induced 'satiety'), adjusting their nutritional patterns and typically experiencing times of frustration or anxiety over perceived nutritional limitations ('low blood sugar, low protein'). Convenient, accessible containers of liquid meal replacements (~300 kcal) will derail the success of the LAGB and frustrate the efforts of the bariatric team.

LAGB Technique

The technical procedure of placing the LAGB should be accessible to all gastrointestinal surgeons appropriately experienced in laparoscopic upper gastrointestinal procedures. Although the technique is typically straightforward and time efficient (typically 30-40 minutes), proctoring and mentoring will ensure that certain technical 'pearls' are learned early and patient safety and outcomes are not compromised. Table 1 gives a summary of the technique.

Patient positioning remains important for LAGB placement despite short procedure times. The patient is typically positioned with arms extended, well padded and secured on standard arm boards attached to operating table. Over extension of the shoulder in these patients is a risk due to challenges with upper extremity size and should be assessed in each patient.

The surgeon may stand on the patient's right if the patient remains supine on the table (recommended) or between the legs for LAGB. If the surgeon is positioned between the legs, either a split leg attachment (maintains patient's hips and knees straight) or stirrups will be necessary.

Careful scrutiny of lower extremity positioning is essential if either of these attachments are used. Pneumatic compression devices are recommended (up to knee or thigh depending on size of lower extremity) regardless of patient positioning. Foley catheters are usually unnecessary, other intra-operative monitoring will be at the discretion of the anesthesia team. If a table mounted liver retractor is used, the appropriate table attachment should be positioned (below right armboard, in line with xiphoid) and secured prior to draping.

Table 1.

Technical Goal	Essential Manoeuvres	Pearls / Potential Pitfalls
Phase 1: Pneumoperitoneum	Subcostal placement of veress needle or open access	Bowel/vascular injury No access: overly lateral positioning due to body habitus
Phase 2: Working ports	Perpendicular trocar placement	Angled placement: restricted instrument movement due to body wall thickness
Phase 3: Mobilize angle of His	Sweep fat pad off diaphragm	Spleen injury
Phase 4: Retrogastric tunnel	Goldfinger passage in retrogastric plane	Landmark: fat pad below right crus Exclude fundus: limit passage of goldfinger
Phase 5: LAGB positioning	Pull LAGB into retrogastric tunnel	Gastric injury: avoid gastric serosa
Phase 6: LAGB closure/suturing	Anterior coverage of LAGB	LAGB damage
Phase 7: Port placement	Securely anchored to abdominal wall	Port migration: expose fascia for secure positioning

Figure 3 shows a typical trocar configuration for the LAGB procedure. The laparscope is inserted two hand breadths below the xiphoid in the midline with a visually guided trocar following veress needle insertion. A 15mm trocar is placed in the left upper quadrant (surgeons right hand, also for LAGB insertion, and position of port) and 5mm working ports are placed in the left flank (assistant) and right upper quadrant (surgeons left hand). A nathanson liver retractor is inserted just to the left of midline at the xiphoid.

Dissection begins by mobilizing the angle of His using a curved dissector or Goldfinger instrument. This sweeping movement separates the fat pad from the diaphragm and creates a target for the tip of the Goldfinger once it is positioned in the retrogastric tunnel.

When this is completed, the pars flaccida is opened and a small fat pad is visualized at the base of the right crus. Dissection is initiated just above this point, only to elevate the posterior aspect of the perigastric fat pad off the retroperitoneum and create a narrow retrogastric tunnel. The dissection should not disrupt the deeper muscular tissues or perigastric fat, instead a plane is created between these two structures. Once the plane is initiated, the Goldfinger instrument is passed behind the stomach and curved into position at the site where the angle of His was mobilized. Limited passage of the Goldfinger will exclude the fundus from the gastric pouch, which is essential to avoid early pouch dilation. Once the Goldfinger is exposed at the angle of His, the LAGB is inserted using the 15mm trocar, attached to the Goldfinger and carefully pulled into position in the retrogastric tunnel. The LAGB is then closed (variable buckle mechanisms exist to close the LAGB) and the anterior aspect is usually covered by suturing gastric tissue over the LAGB to extend the 'tissue tunnel' from posterior to anterior, with the expectation that this will maintain LAGB position.

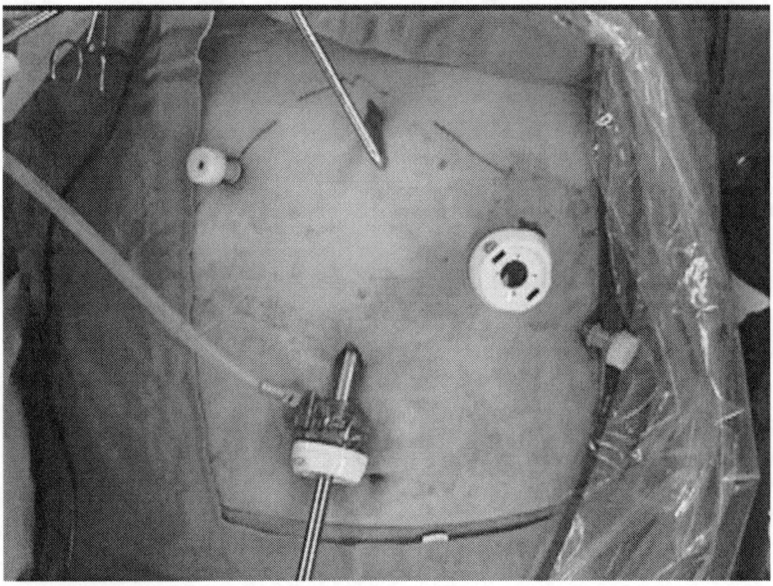

Figure 3. LAGB trocare sites.

Two or three sutures typically secure proximal fundus over the anterior aspect of the band. The tubing is pulled through a trocar and attached to the port device (to be used for band adjustments). Finally, the port is positioned on the abdominal wall (variable positions are used for the port) using either suture or metallic hooks incorporated into the port. Care should be taken to secure the port to the anterior abdominal wall to avoid port migration, this is done by clearing away all subcutaneous fatty tissue. Skin is then closed securely, especially at the port site in order to avoid wound disruption and port extrusion.

Post-Operative Management

Following LAGB, selected patients may be discharged the same day. This may include patients without significant comorbid disease or operative and peri-operative concerns. Typically, patients are discharged the next day, on a limited diet (restricted fluid volumes of approximately 1-1.5L). Patients are seen in early post-operative follow-up at 2-3 weeks to assess for early unexpected complications, meal tolerance and wound healing. The initial LAGB adjustment does not occur until the second visit (4-6 weeks) to allow wound edema and fluid collections around the port to resolve.

The initial LAGB fill is done with a variable amount of normal saline (usually 2 cc). Adjustments may be done in clinic by palpating the port and percutaneously accessing it, or with fluoroscopic guidance. Contrast material can also be given orally to assess changes in restriction if fluoroscopy is used. Subsequent injections of the band are done at 4-6 week intervals, and are based on feedback from dieticians, clinicians and the patient. Untoward symptoms are queried (nausea, vomiting, limited solid intake) and weight loss is determined. Ideally, at the appropriate degree of restriction, the patient is losing .5 – 1.0 kg per week, meal portion sizes are limited to 1-1.5 cups and there are no reports of nausea or vomiting. Patients must be compliant with appropriate meal selection, avoid calorie dense liquids and limit liquids with meals in order to maximize early satiety. Once adequate restriction is achieved, the port does not need to be accessed unless the patient reports a change in restriction (ie with weight loss) or problems arise.

Clinical Outcomes and Complications

At least two systematic reviews have described the satisfactory clinical efficacy of the LAGB. Chapman et al and Obrien et al have show excellent medium term weight loss following LAGB with a favourable safety profile in comparison to more complex procedures. Weight loss of 40-50 percent of excess weight are described. Controversy remains in the surgical community, however regarding the outcomes of the LAGB.

There are concerns of excessive band migration (slip) leading to LAGB removal and treatment failures due to inadequate weight loss. However, lack of standardization of pre-operative patient work-up and comorbid disease screening (mental health), patient selection and follow-up and finally standardized definitions of treatment failure obscure clear interpretation of the literature.

References

Cadière GB, Bruyns J, Himpens J, Favretti F. Laparoscopic gastroplasty for morbid obesity. *Br. J. Surg.* 1994; 81 (10): 1524. PMID 7820493.

Chapman A, Kiroff G, Game P, Foster B, O'Brien P, Ham J, et al. Laparoscopic adjustable gastric banding in the treatment of obesity: A systematic literature review. *Surgery.* 2004;135(3):326-351.

Kuzmak LI. Silicone gastric banding: a simple and effective operation for morbid obesity. *Contemporary Surgery* 1986; 28: 13–8.

O'Brien PE, McPhail T, Chaston TB, Dixon JB. Systematic review of medium-term weight loss after bariatric operations. *Obes Surg.* 2006;16(8):1032-1040.

Suter M, Calmes J, Paroz A, et al. A 10-year experience with laparoscopic gastric banding for morbid obesity: high long-term complication and failure rates. *Obesity Surgery.* 2006;16: 829-835.

Wilkinson LH. Reduction of gastric reservoir capacity. *Am. J. Clin. Nutrition* 1980; 33 (2 Suppl): 515–7. PMID 7355831.

In: The Fundamentals of Bariatric Surgery
Editors: Shahzeer Karmali and Daniel W. Birch
ISBN: 978-1-62417-732-3

Chapter 8

Roux-En-Y Gastric Bypass: Procedure, Mechanism of Action and Outcomes

***Noah J. Switzer*[1], *Kourosh Sarkhosh*[2] and *Shahzeer Karmali*[2,3]**
[1]Faculty of Medicine and Dentistry, University of Alberta, Edmonton, Alberta, Canada
[2]Center for the Advancement of Minimally Invasive Surgery (CAMIS), Royal Alexandria Hospital, Edmonton, Alberta, Canada
[3]Department of Surgery, University of Alberta, Edmonton, Alberta, Canada

Abstract

The Roux-en-Y Gastric Bypass (RYGB) is one of the most common abdominal procedures performed in North America. This bariatric procedure involves altering the normal digestive tract anatomy through a reduction in the total stomach volume and the creation of two separate limbs, the roux and biliopancreatic. This enables the nutrients flowing through the tract to bypass part of the intestine. The standard of practice is to perform the bypass laparoscopically versus open, as this results in reductions in post-operative wound infections, hospital stay and post-operative pain scores. RYGB has an irreversible mechanism of action that is both restrictive and malabsorptive, decreasing both the oral intake and limiting the re-absorption of nutrients. However, the alterations in specific gut hormones (ghrelin, incretins, and PYY) are starting to become recognized as the key contributor to its clinical efficacy. The outcomes for patients post-procedure are drastic. Most studies report an excess weight loss (EWL) of 60-70%; with the maintenance of this weight loss reported almost a decade after surgery. It is important to recognize that this impressive weight loss cannot be replicated by merely pharmaceutical, diet or lifestyle regimens. The improvement in comorbid conditions is also part of what makes RYGB such a successful procedure. Within 3 days of their RYGB, 30% of diabetic patients will be discharged free of their anti-diabetes medication, with complete resolution of their diabetes seen in over 80% of patients. Other comorbidities also significantly improve following RYGB, such as hypertension, hyperlipidemia, and obstructive sleep apnea.

There is also a modest decrease in mortality rate with surgically managed patients compared to controls. In conclusion, due to it its significant weight loss and improvement in comorbid conditions, the Roux-en-Y gastric bypass is a reliable and proven weight loss strategy for the morbidly obese.

Introduction

Since Mason and Ito performed the first reported gastric bypass in 1967, it has grown to become one of the most common abdominal procedures in Canada and the United States. [1, 2] Of the bariatric procedures available, the gastric bypass is the most studied and arguably the most successful, in terms of weight loss, and improvement of co-morbid conditions. The procedure involves decreasing the size of the stomach and recreating the normal flow of nutrients. The literature states an average weight loss of 60-70% of excess weight with a greater than 80% resolution in diabetes, hyperlipidemia, hypertension and obstructive sleep apnea [3]. In this review, we examine the Roux-en-Y gastric bypass (RYGB) as a technical procedure, its mechanism of action and its efficacy in producing significant weight loss and improving obesity-related comorbidities.

Procedure

Generally, the RYGB involves disrupting digestive continuity by dividing the stomach into two unequal parts. Nutrients flow from the oral cavity into a small gastric pouch (approximately 5% of the total stomach size) and outlet though a portion of distal jejunum referred to as the roux or alimentary limb [2, 4]. The gastric, bile and pancreatic secretions are transmitted through the larger distal end of the stomach or proximal small intestine and flow down the biliopancreatic limb. These two limbs eventually anastomose downstream at the jejunojejunostomy. The Roux-en-Y bypass is favored over traditional one-anastomosis bypasses, like the loop gastric bypass, due to the fact that it decreases the tension on the gastrojejunostomy and it reduces the reflux of secretions from the pancreas and liver upward into the esophagus and stomach [2] (Figure 1). In brief, the patient is placed in a supine position on the operating table, and either a midline or port incision is made to enter the peritoneal cavity. The ligament of Trietz is then identified at the base of the transverse colon mesentery, which is a major procedural landmark [5].

Once identified, the small bowel is followed 30-40 cm distally where the biliopancreatic limb is created by dividing the jejunum and mobilizing its mesentery [6] The jejunum is then followed an additional 100 cm distally to form the roux limb, for a standard length gastric bypass, to where the jejunojejunostomy will be created in a side to side fashion using a linear stapler. After this, it is important to close the inter-mesenteric defect to prevent the complication of an internal hernia [7].

Next, the greater omentrum is then divided roughly at midline and roux limb is brought up in an ante-colic fashion towards the stomach. To create the gastric pouch, a small window is made in the lesser omentum, and a cutting stapler is entered and fired perpendicular to the lesser curvature of the stomach. With the help of the anesthesiologist, a 50 French bougie is inserted into the oropharynx and down into the stomach.

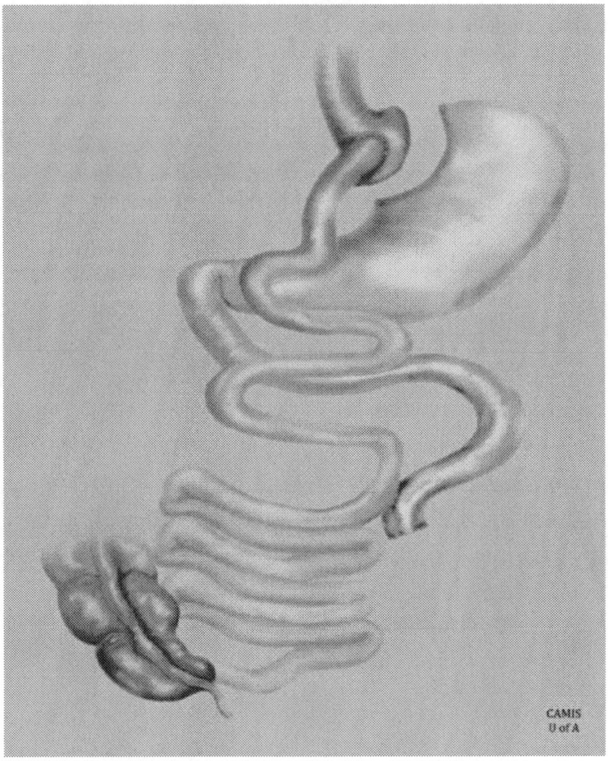

Figure 1.

This bougie will provide the outline for the gastric pouch formation, usually 15-30 mL in total volume, and its best placement is approximately 5-7 cm distal to the esophogastric junction [5] With the bougie in place, between 4-6 more firings of the cutting stapler are used to form the gastric pouch . The exact dimensions of the pouch are highly variable to each institution, but the fundus is usually excluded [2, 5].

The next step is the creation of the gastrojejunostomy, using the circular anastomosis (EEA) technique [6]. To do this, with the help of the anesthesiologist, a 21 or 25 mm Orvil is passed orally down into the gastric pouch. This is brought out of the stomach in an ante-gastric fashion. The jejunal-roux limb is brought up close to the pouch and opened parallel to the staple line. A circular stapler is inserted into the abdominal cavity and into the small bowel lumen and brought out through its antimesenteric side. The Orvil and circular stapler are then mated, the stapler is closed and fired [5, 6]. By doing so, an end to side anastomosis is fashioned between the gastric pouch and jejunum. Jejunal defect is subsequently closed with a stapler.

Prior to closure of the wound and exiting the peritoneal cavity, a gastroscope is inserted to visualize the gastrojejunostomy and to inspect for any leaks; this is done through insufflation of gastric pouch with air and subsequent injection of methylene blue dye intra-luminally and inspecting the anastomosis laparoscopically for any leaks [6].

An upper gastrointestinal study is also performed in postoperative day 1 to rule out any leaks. Typically patients are discharged home on postoperative day 2 on a full fluid diet. A normal diet is initiated usually in 4 weeks time.

The procedure detailed is how the RYGB is performed at our institution, but we acknowledge that there can be differences in the surgical technique. One possible point of difference relates to the ante-colic versus retro-colic placement of the gastrojejunostomy. Liu et al. performed a study comparing these two techniques and found no significant difference in short-term outcomes [8] The second point of possible variation lies in the use of the circular stapler versus the linear stapler and the hand-sewn technique to create the gastrojejunostomy.

Studies have shown that there is no significant difference in the rate of anastomotic leak between the three groups [9]. There may be, however, a reduced risk of an anastomosis stricture with the use of the linear stapler compared to the circular stapler [10, 11].

The standard of practice is to perform the RYGB laparoscopically versus open. This is attributed to the reductions in post-operative wound infections, hospital stay and post-operative pain scores experienced by patients post-minimally invasive surgery [6].

Laparoscopic intervention is especially advantageous in high risk populations (multiple comorbidities) due to their particular vulnerability to cardiopulmonary and wound related complications.[6] It is important to recognize that the gastric bypass is a complicated procedure with a steep technical learning curve. Maggard et al. reported that mortality rates decrease from 6% to nearly 0% for surgeons with over 250 procedures of experience and leak rates drop from 3% to 1% for veteran surgeons of at least 300 procedures [1].

Mechanism of Action

Traditionally, the mechanism behind bariatric operations is classified as either restrictive or malabsorptive. Restrictive procedures manipulate the functional volume of the stomach thereby limiting the amount of oral intake, while malabsorptive procedures limit the amount of digestion and re-absorption that takes place in the stomach and small intestine due to the re-routing of nutrients [2].

RYGB is an irreversible hybrid of both of these. However, recent studies have failed to show any significant malabsorption of fat, cholesterol, or carbohydrates following RYGB and are not linking any sub-significant malabsorption to noteworthy weight loss [4, 12].

This leads to the growing awareness of another mechanism playing an important role, the gut hormones (ghrelin, incretins, and PYY) and the decreasing utility of the old classification.

Ghrelin

Ghrelin is an orexigenic gut hormone that stimulates appetite and modulates satiety. Following RYGB, ghrelin levels are reduced, most likely to due manipulation of the gastric fundus; which is responsible for ghrelin secretion [12]. As a result, the patient feels a reduction in their hunger drive, decreasing their oral intake. The long-term alterations in ghrelin levels are still not fully understood, as there are studies reporting the rise of long-term ghrelin levels, while other studies report the contrary [12].

Incretins

Incretins are gut hormones that augment the release of insulin and promote pancreatic beta cell proliferation [12, 13]. Incretins, glucose-dependent insulinotropic polypeptide (GIP) and glucagon-like peptide 1 (GLP-1), are responsible for approximately 50% of insulin release following meals [14] They are also responsible for promoting weight loss, appetite suppression, and increasing hepatic and muscle insulin sensitivity [14]. After RYGB, circulating levels of post-prandial GLP-1 are enhanced 5-10 fold, which is correlated to an improvement in glucose homeostasis [14] There are a few theories of why this enhancement phenomenon exists.

The foregut hypothesis states that nutrients being shunted from the duodenal benefits glucose tolerance, while the hindgut hypothesis states that the rapid exposure of nutrients to the distal ileum causes the spiked levels of incretins after a meal [14] Long term data on incretin levels post RYGB report that this enhancement of incretin release persists over time. One study even reported elevated GLP-1 and GIP levels 20 years later [14].

PPY

Peptide YY (PYY) is an appetite suppressant gut hormone, whose blunted, pathological dysfunction is documented in obesity. Literature states as early as day 2 following RYGB, PYY levels are increased upwards of 10-fold [12] Patients no longer experience the exaggerated hunger craves that they had before surgery, probably due to the re-routing of nutrients from the stomach to the distal jejunum [12].

Outcomes

Weight Change

The main objective of any bariatric operation is to produce significant weight loss. After RYGB, most studies report an excess weight loss (EWL) of 60-70%. [6] Buchwald et al. detailed a mean EWL of 68.2% in 2742 patients, corresponding to an initial weight loss of almost 35%. [3]

Similar figures were reported by Maggard et al. in their meta-analysis; they found a mean 1-year weight loss following RYGB of 43.5 kg in 2937 patients, with no significant difference between open versus laparoscopic groups [1] They also compared weight loss from surgery to that of pharmaceutical, diet and lifestyle regimens and reported the superiority of surgery over these over groups, especially with patients with body mass index (BMI) greater than 40 where this difference is of an order of magnitude [1].

The maintenance of this weight loss has also been reported. A 7-year retrospective study reported a 5-year post RYGB absolute weight loss of 34.5 kg. [15] There is however evidence of minor but significant long-term weight regain. There are a number mechanisms postulated to be responsible from gastric pouch dilatation, decrease in energy expenditure (exercise), decrease in metabolism, to return of gut hormones back to pre-surgical levels [16].

Type 2 Diabetes Mellitus

The resolution of diabetes after RYGB appears to be weight independent as it usually occurs within a few weeks before any appreciable weight loss can occur [13] Buchwald et al. reported an improvement in diabetes for 93.2% of patients after RYGB, with a complete resolution of their diabetes in 83.7%. [3] This coincided with a reduction in HbA_{1c}, fasting glucose and fasting insulin of 0.59%, 1.25 mmol/L and121.26 mmol/L respectively.[3] As stated earlier, this improvement can be quite dramatic, as within 3 days of their RYGB, 30% of diabetic patients will be discharged free of their anti-diabetes medication and with plasma glucose levels within the normal range [13] These patients are expected to remain eugylcemic in the long-term, with literature reporting maintained diabetic resolution after 14 years post-operation [13] It is once again important to note that the degree of normalization of glucose homeostasis seen after RYGB cannot be replicated by pharmaceutical or lifestyle regimens (diet and exercise) [13].

Interestingly, the dramatic success of RYGB on the resolution of diabetes has spawned the operation being relabeled as a "metabolic gastric bypass," where diabetic patients, with BMIs as low as 22, undergo this procedure for curative intent of their diabetes. This practice however is quite controversial and is not being recommended for diabetics with BMIs under 30 [13].

Hypertension, Hyperlipidemia, Obstructive Sleep Apnea (OSA)

Other comorbidities also significantly improve following RYGB. Ahmed et al. followed 100 patients prospectively after RYGB and reported an early mean reduction in systolic (9 mmHg) and diastolic (7 mmHg) blood pressures within the first week and a reduction in the total anti-hypertensive medication usage by one-third from pre-surgery levels [17] Overall, 87.2% of patients will see an improvement in their high blood pressure; with 67.5% of patients experiencing a complete resolution of their hypertension [3].

Greater than 90% of patients with hyperlipidemia, hypercholesterolemia, and hypertriglyceridemia experienced an improvement in their pathologic lipid levels. This corresponded to a significant reduction in total cholesterol, low-density lipoprotein and triglyceride levels of 0.96, 0.89, and 1.07 respectively [3]. In a retrospective study of 100 patients, at 6-month follow up after RYGB, most patients did not require lipid lower agents, and remarkably, by the end of the study, all patients were off their anti-hyperlipidemia agents [18] Obstructive sleep apnea (OSA) is a common comorbidity in the severely obese population, affecting 44% of all bariatric surgical patients [19] Following RYGB, 94.8% of these patients are expected to see an improvement in their OSA, with 80.4% having complete resolution [3] This corresponds to improvement in arterial blood gases, respiratory tests and polysomnographic studies, as well as a reduction in the apnea-hypopnea index [19, 20].

Mortality

There is growing evidence that, in comparison to similarly obese patients who are medically managed, surgically managed patients, through RYGB, have a modest decrease in mortality rate [16]. A multicentre study in Sweden, known as the SOS study, and a 20 000 patient study in Utah found a long-term mortality benefit in surgical patients versus matched obese patients [13] More specifically, in their Utah study, Adams et al. described a 40% reduction in cause-specific mortality; this was stratified into coronary artery disease (56% reduction), diabetes (92% reduction), and cancer (60% reduction). [21] Furthermore, Donadelli et al. reported a significant reduction in the 10-year cardiovascular risk for RYGB patients after their surgery, using the Framingham risk score, as early as 2 years following their surgical intervention [22].

Conclusion

The RYGB is the most common bariatric procedure performed in North America [2] Its documented success in resolving the metabolic syndrome has been attributed to many mechanisms, such as restriction and malabsorption of nutrients and alterations of the gut hormone levels [13] It remains a complicated procedure with a steep learning curve, but it provides an excess weight loss that cannot be paralleled by pharmaceutical or lifestyle regimes or most other bariatric operations [3] In conclusion, the success of the Roux-en-Y gastric bypass makes it an efficacious option for the morbidly obese patient with multiple comorbidities.

References

[1] Maggard MA, Shugarman LR, Suttorp M, Maglione M, Sugerman HJ, Livingston EH, Nguyen NT, Li Z, Mojica WA, Hilton L, Rhodes S, Morton SC, Shekelle PG. Meta-analysis: Surgical treatment of obesity. *Ann. Intern. Med.* 2005;142:547-559.

[2] Herron DM, Roohipour R. Bariatric surgical anatomy and mechanisms of action. *Gastrointest Endosc. Clin. N Am.* 2011;21:213-228.

[3] Buchwald H, Avidor Y, Braunwald E, Jensen MD, Pories W, Fahrbach K, Schoelles K. Bariatric surgery: A systematic review and meta-analysis. *JAMA.* 2004;292:1724-1737.

[4] Brolin RE. Bariatric surgery and long-term control of morbid obesity. *JAMA.* 2002;288:2793-2796.

[5] Townsend C, Evers B. *Atlas of general surgery techniques*. Saunders Elsevier; 2010.

[6] Schauer PR, Ikramuddin S, Gourash W, Ramanathan R, Luketich J. Outcomes after laparoscopic roux-en-y gastric bypass for morbid obesity. *Ann. Surg.* 2000;232: 515-529.

[7] Aghajani E, Jacobsen HJ, Nergaard BJ, Hedenbro JL, Leifson BG, Gislason H. Internal hernia after gastric bypass: A new and simplified technique for laparoscopic primary closure of the mesenteric defects. *J Gastrointest Surg*. 2012;16:641-645.

[8] Liu XM, Wang CC, Hu YZ, Yang JG, Huang J, Ding H, Li JY, Pan YL, Shen YY, Yu CL, Yu HB. [antecolic versus retrocolic gastroenteric anastomosis for laparoscopic roux-en-y gastric bypass: A prospective randomized control trial]. *Zhonghua Wei Chang Wai Ke Za Zhi*. 2011;14:422-424.

[9] Finks JF, Carlin A, Share D, O'Reilly A, Fan Z, Birkmeyer J, Birkmeyer N, Michigan Bariatric Surgery Collaborative from the Michigan Surgical Collaborative for Outcomes Research E. Effect of surgical techniques on clinical outcomes after laparoscopic gastric bypass--results from the michigan bariatric surgery collaborative. *Surg. Obes. Relat. Dis*. 2011;7:284-289.

[10] Giordano S, Salminen P, Biancari F, Victorzon M. Linear stapler technique may be safer than circular in gastrojejunal anastomosis for laparoscopic roux-en-y gastric bypass: A meta-analysis of comparative studies. *Obes. Surg*. 2011;21:1958-1964.

[11] Leyba JL, Llopis SN, Isaac J, Aulestia SN, Bravo C, Obregon F. Laparoscopic gastric bypass for morbid obesity-a randomized controlled trial comparing two gastrojejunal anastomosis techniques. *JSLS*. 2008;12:385-388.

[12] Scott WR, Batterham RL. Roux-en-y gastric bypass and laparoscopic sleeve gastrectomy: Understanding weight loss and improvements in type 2 diabetes after bariatric surgery. *Am J Physiol Regul Integr Comp Physiol*. 2011;301:R15-27.

[13] Ashrafian H, Athanasiou T, Li JV, Bueter M, Ahmed K, Nagpal K, Holmes E, Darzi A, Bloom SR. Diabetes resolution and hyperinsulinaemia after metabolic roux-en-y gastric bypass. *Obes Rev*. 2011;12:e257-272.

[14] Laferrere B. Do we really know why diabetes remits after gastric bypass surgery? *Endocrine*. 2011;40:162-167.

[15] Smith SC, Goodman GN, Edwards CB. Roux-en-y gastric bypass: A 7-year retrospective review of 3,855 patients. *Obes. Surg*. 1995;5:314-318.

[16] Shah M, Simha V, Garg A. Review: Long-term impact of bariatric surgery on body weight, comorbidities, and nutritional status. *J Clin Endocrinol Metab*. 2006;91:4223-4231.

[17] Ahmed AR, Rickards G, Coniglio D, Xia Y, Johnson J, Boss T, O'Malley W. Laparoscopic roux-en-y gastric bypass and its early effect on blood pressure. *Obes. Surg*. 2009;19:845-849.

[18] Jamal M, Wegner R, Heitshusen D, Liao J, Samuel I. Resolution of hyperlipidemia follows surgical weight loss in patients undergoing roux-en-y gastric bypass surgery: A 6-year analysis of data. *Surg. Obes. Relat Dis*. 2011;7:473-479.

[19] Marti-Valeri C, Sabate A, Masdevall C, Dalmau A. Improvement of associated respiratory problems in morbidly obese patients after open roux-en-y gastric bypass. *Obes. Surg*. 2007;17:1102-1110.

[20] Fritscher LG, Canani S, Mottin CC, Fritscher CC, Berleze D, Chapman K, Chatkin JM. Bariatric surgery in the treatment of obstructive sleep apnea in morbidly obese patients. *Respiration*. 2007;74:647-652.

[21] Adams TD, Gress RE, Smith SC, Halverson RC, Simper SC, Rosamond WD, Lamonte MJ, Stroup AM, Hunt SC. Long-term mortality after gastric bypass surgery. *N. Engl. J. Med*. 2007;357:753-761.

[22] Donadelli SP, Salgado W, Jr., Marchini JS, Schmidt A, Amato CA, Ceneviva R, Dos Santos JE, Nonino CB. Change in predicted 10-year cardiovascular risk following roux-en-y gastric bypass surgery: Who benefits? *Obes. Surg*. 2011;21:569-573.

In: The Fundamentals of Bariatric Surgery
Editors: Shahzeer Karmali and Daniel W. Birch
ISBN: 978-1-62417-732-3

Chapter 9

Biliopancreatic Diversion with Duodenal Switch

Usmaan Hameed[1] and Allan Okrainec[1,2]
[1] Division of General Surgery, University of Toronto, Toronto, Canada
[2]University Health Network in Toronto, Canada

History

In 1954, Kremen's trial of a surgical weight loss strategy described bypassing the majority of the small bowel by anastomosing the proximal jejunum to the distal ileum [1] (Figure 1). However, JIB had significant complications such as blind loop syndrome in the defunctioned limb, abdominal bloating, migratory arthralgias and liver dysfunction. Patients who underwent JIB also exhibited severe malabsorptive difficulties including protein depletion, severe diarrhea, electrolyte abnormality, vitamin deficiency, nephropathy, and cirrhosis.

Scopinaro first described the classic biliopancreatic diversion in 1979 as an alternative to the JIB [3]. The BPD included a distal gastrectomy, a 200cm Roux limb and 50cm common channel (Figure 2). Patients had significant long-term weight loss, but also experienced significant side effects including: stomal ulceration; diarrhea, foul smelling stool and flatulence related to dumping syndrome; and malabsorptive sequelae such as anemia, protein malnutrition, peripheral neuropathy, Wernicke's encephalopathy, and bone demineralization [4].

In 1987 Demeester described the 'duodenal switch' (DS), or suprapapillary duodenojejunostomy, which was sought as an alternative technique to Roux-en-y biliary diversion in patients with bile alkaline gastritis. His experimental work performed on dogs (Figure 3) shows that preserving a short segment of proximal duodenum (Groups C and D) yields lower rates of ulceration while preserving weight loss in those that have undergone jejunoileal bypass (Groups A and C). In his clinical results, patients undergoing DS would have improved gastric emptying, reduced symptoms of alkaline reflux and lower rates of jejunal ulcers than those undergoing classical Roux-en-y [5].

The biliopancreatic diversion with duodenal switch (BPD-DS) was described independently in 1998 by Hess and Hess, and by Marceau as a hybrid of Scopinaro's BPD and Demeester's DS with the goal of achieving sustainable weight loss without the associated malabsorptive morbidity.

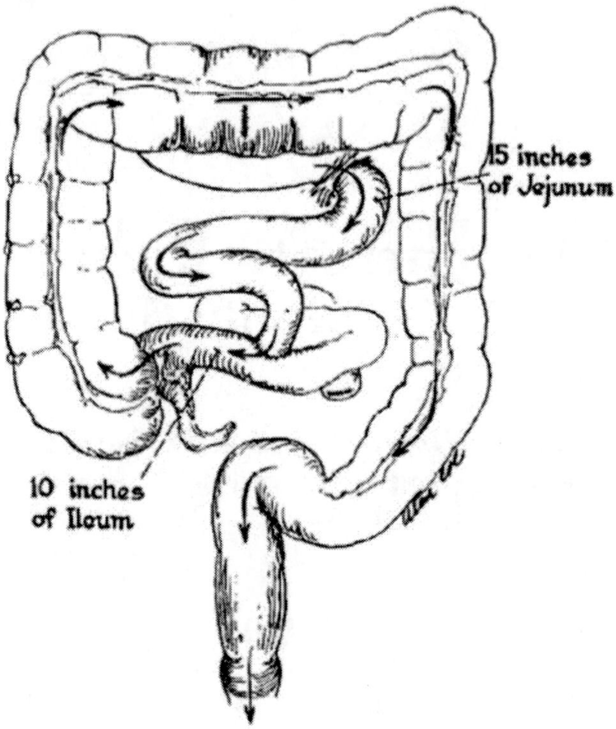

Figure 1. Jejunoileal Bypass [2].

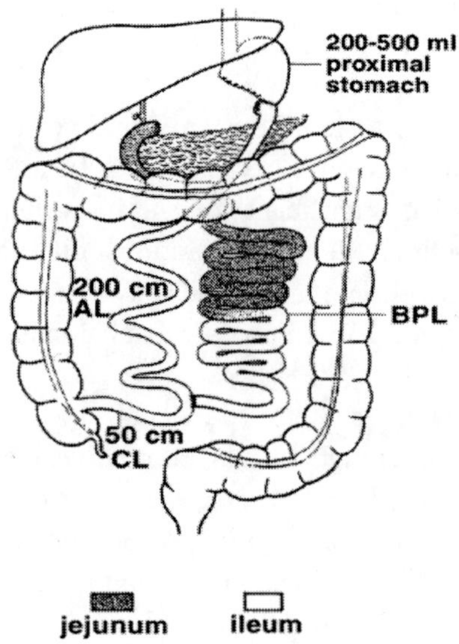

Figure 2. Biliopancreatic Bypass [4].

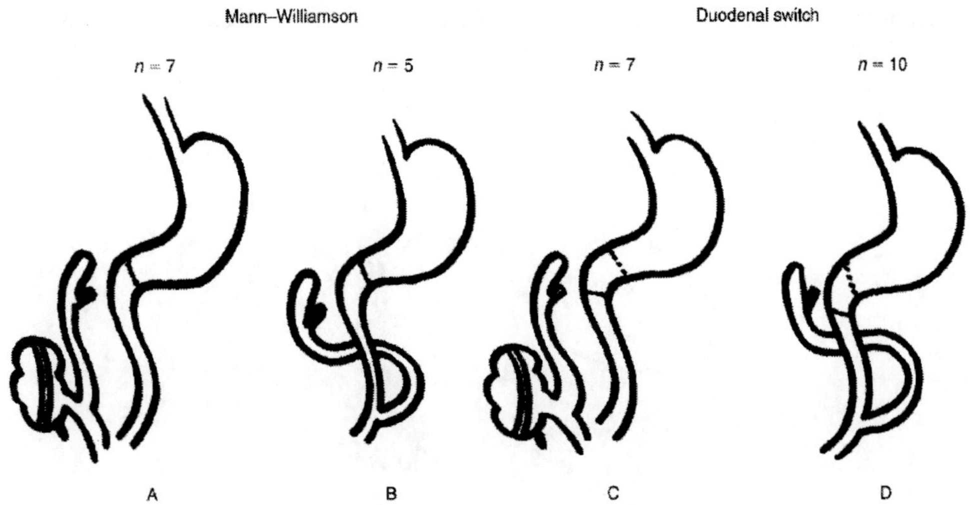

	A	B	C	D
Ulcer*	86% (6/7)	100% (5/5)	29% (2/7)	10% (1/10)
Perforation	43% (3/7)	60% (3/5)	14% (1/7)	0% (0/10)
Weight loss	33%	7%	33%	5%
Follow-up	3 months	3 months	3 months	1 year

*A vs C $P = 0.05$ B vs D $P = 0.002$ A vs D $P = 0.003$

Figure 3. Demeester's experiment in dogs show that preserving the pylorus and proximal duodenum is protective against stomal ulcers. Those that underwent jejunoileal bypass (Groups A and C) also maintained their weight loss when the pylorus and duodenum were preserved [5].

Technique

The technique described by Hess customizes the malabsorptive component to each patient by first measuring the distance from the ligament of Treitz to the terminal ileum (Figure 4) [6,7]. The length of the alimentary limb is calculated by multiplying the total length of the small bowel by 40%. The common channel is 10% of the small bowel length, encompassing the distal portion of the alimentary limb to the terminal ileum. Each site is marked with a stitch. The alimentary limb, which includes the Roux and common channel, is approximately 250-335 cm in length. The result is a common channel between 75-100cm in length; approximately 25-50 cm longer than the 50cm of the classic BPD. Surgeons that use fixed lengths typically use a common channel of 75cm and alimentary limb of 250cm [8].

Rather than performing a distal gastrectomy as in the classic BPD, the pylorus is preserved and the greater curvature of the stomach resected in a sleeve configuration for the restrictive component of the surgery. The short gastric vessels are divided from approximately 5 cm distal to the pylorus to the esophagus along the greater curvature.

A penrose drain is passed around the first part of the duodenum. A 40F dilator is used to size the sleeve, which is created using several firings of the linear stapler. The duodenum is transected 4-5 cm distal to the pylorus. The stomach is then filled with saline and methylene blue to check for leaks and measure the stomach volume. Hess and Vage describe best weight loss results with an ideal stomach volume of 90-120ml [6,9]. The duodenoileal retrocolic end-to-end anastomosis and ileo-ileal end-to-side anastomosis are then performed and mesenteric defects are closed.

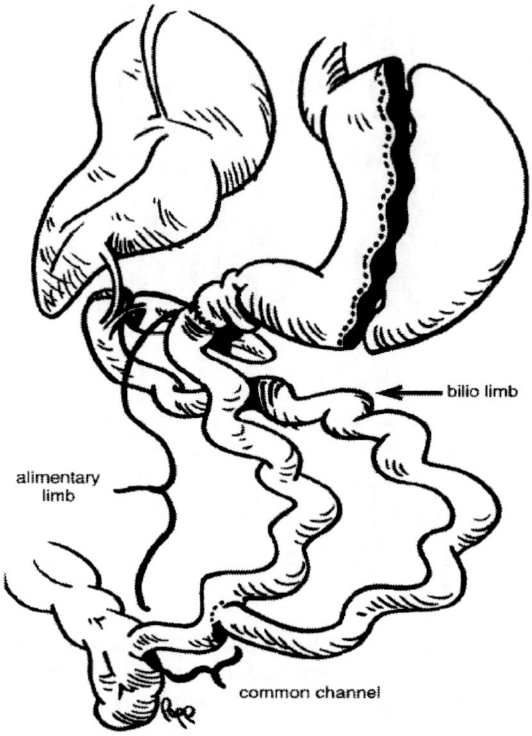

Figure 4. Biliopancreatic Diversion with Duodenal Switch [6].

There are several variations to the approach described by Hess, including 2-staged approaches beginning with the gastric sleeve as the initial stage and the BPD-DS as the second stage [10]. Patients with a BMI of >60 have been reported to have a perioperative mortality as high as 6.5%. [11] This may support a staged approach, however several studies have described low mortality rates with single-staged BPD-DS in patients with BMI>50. [12] Alternatives in anastomotic techniques such as performing an end-to-side duodenoileal anastomoses, hand sewn versus stapled techniques, and variations in the alimentary and common channel lengths have also been described. [8, 13].

The laparoscopic BPD-DS, first described by Gagner and Ren in 2000, is gaining popularity with increasing familiarity with advanced laparoscopy in bariatric patients and is now the most popular approach to this procedure. [14, 15] The technical complexity of the surgery and longer operative times are the main factors limiting laparoscopy. However, decreased postoperative pain, length of stay, and wound complications such as infection and incisional hernia make this an attractive technique. Robotic approaches have also been explored largely in revisional surgery, such as converting failed laparoscopic gastric bands or bypass to BPD-DS. [16].

Indications

BPD-DS was originally described as revisional surgery for those who had failed gastric banding or gastroplasty [6] Goals of aggressive weight loss in superobese patients with a BMI > 50 and revisional surgery are the most common indications for patients undergoing BPD-DS. [17] Good results have also been shown in patients with a BMI<50 with similar rates of perioperative morbidity, although the long term risks of vitamin deficiencies and protein depletion in these patients must be factored in. Hess advocates that BPD-DS should be the gold standard for bariatric patients, however this topic remains controversial due to the risk of malabsorption [18].

Outcomes

Weight loss data in BPD-DS are amongst the highest described of any bariatric surgical procedure. In his 10-year review on 161 patients, Hess described an average excess weight loss up to 74%, with 95% of patients having EWL% of greater than 50%. [19].

Resolution of obesity-related comorbidities such as type II diabetes, hypertension hypercholesterolemia, obstructive sleep apnea have been shown in most studies to be superior with BPD-DS than with RYGB. [20, 21] A randomized control trial comparing BPD-DS and RYGB by described improved 1-year weight loss in the BPD-DS group with comparable perioperative morbidity and mortality, but longer operative time and length of stay. Crea demonstrated that 99% of patients undergoing BPD-DS had either resolution or improvement in their hypertension, hypercholesterolemia and diabetes and 98% percent of diabetics who were previously on oral hypoglycemic agents had stopped their medications within 1 year of surgery [22].

Physiology

The exact mechanism for weight loss and reduction in comorbidities after biliopancreatic diversion with duodenal switch is unknown, however more is known now then ever before. BPD-DS has a restrictive as well as malabsorptive component contributing to weight loss. Most of the early weight loss is thought to be due to gastric restriction, whereas sustained long-term weight loss is thought to be secondary to the malabsorptive component of the diversion.

Gastric restriction mechanically limits the volume of food intake due to the size of the stomach after vertical sleeve gastrectomy. As mentioned above, the ideal stomach volumes are estimated at 90-120ml. The goal is to balance intake restriction with the risk of inadequate protein and caloric intake, which may be seen if the stomach is made too small.

Sustained weight loss is mainly determined by the degree of lipid malabsorption. The length of the common channel directly affects lipid absorption. With shorter common channels, lipids do not have enough surface area or transit time to be absorbed. With longer common channels, the lipid absorption may be too great, and weight loss may be hindered. The length of the alimentary channel similarly affects protein absorption. In the BPD-DS, the patient risks protein deficiency should the alimentary limb be constructed too short, and may require future revision. The alimentary limb length affects carbohydrate absorption, although to a much lesser degree than protein absorption. Even still, levels of fasting glucose and insulin are significantly lower in patients who underwent BPD-DS compared to patients of lower BMI who had not undergone surgery [23].

Gastric emptying also appears to be more rapid in BPD-DS patients compared to patients with RYGB or gastric band, however is not commonly associated with dumping as the previous BPD with distal gastrectomy. As a result of the faster transit, anorexigenic peptides PYY are released and are found to be in higher circulating levels in BPD-DS patients. PYY and GLP-1 are thought to be among the factors contributing to early satiety [24].

References

[1] Kremen A, Linner J, Nelson C. An experimental evaluation of the nutritional importance of proximal and distal small intestine. *Ann. Surg.* 1954;140:439–44.

[2] Payne J, DeWind L, Commons R. Metabolic observations in patients with jejunocolic shunts. *Am. J. Surg.* 1963;106:273–89.

[3] Scopinaro N, Gianetta E, Civalleri D, et al. Bilio-pancreatic by-pass for obesity: II. Initial experience in man. *Br. J. Surg.* 1979;66:619–20.

[4] Scopinaro N, Gianetti E, Adami G, et al. Biliopancreatic diversion for obesity at eighteen years. *Surgery* 1996;119:261–8.

[5] DeMeester T, Fuchs K, Ball C, et al. Experimental and clinical results with proximal end-to-end duodenojejunostomy for the pathologic duodenogastric reflux. *Ann. Surg.* 1987;206:414–24.

[6] Hess DS, Hess DW. Biliopancreatic diversion with a duodenal switch. *Obes. Surg.* 1998;8:267–82.

[7] Lagace M, Marceau P, Marceau S, et al. Biliopancreatic diversion with a new type of gastrectomy: some previous conclusions revisited. *Obes Surg.* 1995;5:411–8.

[8] Scopinaro N. Thirty-Five Years of Biliopancreatic Diversion: Notes on Gastrointestinal Physiology to Complete the Published Information Useful for a Better Understanding and Clinical Use of the Operation. *Obes. Surg.* 2012;22:427-432.

[9] Våge V, Gåsdal CG, Laukland C et al. The Biliopancreatic Diversion with a Duodenal Switch (BPDDS): How is it Optimally Performed? *Obes Surg.* 2011;21;1864-1869.

[10] Dapri G, Cadiere GB, Himpens J. Superobese and Super-superobese patients: 2-step laparoscopic duodenal switch. *Surg Obes Relat Dis.* 2011; 7; 703-708.

[11] Kim WW, Gagner M, Kini S, et al. Laparoscopic vs. open biliopancreatic diversion with duodenal switch: a comparative study. *J. Gastrointest Surg.* 2003;7(4):552–7.

[12] Topart P, Becouarn G, Ritz P. Should biliopancreatic diversion with duodenal switch be done as single-stage procedure in patients with BMI _50 kg/m2? *Surg.Obes. Relat Dis.* 2010;6;59-63.

[13] Baltasar A. Hand-sewn laparoscopic duodenal switch. *Surg. Obes. Relat Dis.* 2007;3(1):94–6.

[14] Ren CJ, Patterson E, Gagner M. Early results of laparoscopic biliopancreatic diversion with duodenal switch: a case series of 40 consecutive patients. *Obes. Surg.* 2000; 10: 514–523.

[15] Ramos AC, Galvao Neto M, Santana Galvao M, et al. Simplified laparoscopic duodenal switch. *Surg. Obes. Relat Dis* 2007;3(5):565–8.

[16] Sudan R, Puri V, Sudan D. Robotically assisted biliary pancreatic diversion with a duodenal switch: a new technique. *Surg. Endosc.* 2007;21(5):729–33.

[17] Hess DS. Biliopancreatic diversion with duodenal switch. 2004 ASBS Consensus Conference. Surg Obes Relat Dis. 2005;1: 329–333.

[18] Biertho L, Biron S, Marceau P et al. Is biliopancreatic diversion with duodenal switch indicated for patients with body mass index >50 kg/m2? SOARD. 2010;6:508–515.

[19] Hess DS, Hess DW, Oakley RS. The Biliopancreatic diversion with the duodenal switch: results beyond 10 years. *Obes. Surg.* 2005. 15;408-416.

[20] Prachand VS, Ward M, Alverdy JC. Duodenal switch provides superior resolution of metabolic comorbidities independent of weight loss in the super-obese (BMI≥50 kg/m2) compared with gastric bypass. *J.* Gastrointest Surg. 2010. 14:211–220.

[21] Prachand VN, DaVee RT, Alverdy JC. Duodenal switch provides superior weight loss in the super-obese (BMI≥50 kg/m2) compared with gastric bypass. *Ann. Surg.* 2006;244:611–619.

[22] Crea N, Pata G, Mittempergher F. Long-Term Results of Biliopancreatic Diversion with or Without Gastric Preservation for Morbid Obesity. *Obes. Surg.* 2011. 21: 139–145.

[23] Johanssen HE, Haenni A, Zethelius B. Bileopancreatic diversion with duodenal switch lowers both early and late phases of glucose, insulin. *Obes. Surg.* 2010. 20:549–558. and proinsulin Responses After Meal. *Obes. Surg.* 2010. 20:549–558.

[24] Hedberg J, Hedenstrom H, Sundbom M. Gastric emptying and postprandial PYY response after biliopancreatic diversion with duodenal switch. *Obes. Surg.* 2011.21:609–615.

In: The Fundamentals of Bariatric Surgery
Editors: Shahzeer Karmali and Daniel W. Birch
ISBN: 978-1-62417-732-3

Chapter 10

Sleeve Gastrectomy: Procedure, Mechanism of Action and Outcomes

Richdeep S. Gill[1], Kevin A. Whitlock[2], David Al-Adra[1], Daniel W. Birch[3] and Shahzeer Karmali[1,3]
[1]Department of Surgery, University of Alberta, Edmonton, Alberta, Canada
[2]Faculty of Medicine and Dentistry, University of Alberta, Edmonton, Alberta, Canada
[3]Center for the Advancement of Minimally Invasive Surgery (CAMIS), Royal Alexandria Hospital, Edmonton, Alberta, Canada

Abstract

Globally, an estimated 300 million adults are considered clinically obese. Obesity is associated with multiple co-morbidities including type-2 diabetes mellitus (T2DM) and hypertension. Bariatric surgery, as part of a comprehensive weight management strategy has been shown to produce marked weight loss and improvement of co-morbidities. While laparoscopic sleeve gastrectomy (LSG), initially introduced as the first procedure in a two-staged approach for high-risk super-obese patients, it has emerged as an important stand alone surgical option. LSG is typically classified as primarily restrictive procedure, however recent evidence suggests that it performs better than other restrictive procedures, in terms of weight loss and T2DM remission. The procedure involves creation of a gastric tube with approximate capacity of 60 - 100 mL. In this review, we explore LSG as a technical procedure, its mechanism of action and its effectiveness in producing weight loss and improving obesity-related comorbidities.

Introduction

Over the past 30 years there has been an increase in the average body mass index (BMI) worldwide [1]. As a result, over 20% of the world's population are considered overweight and

10% are defined as clinically obese (BMI ≥30 kg/m^2) [2]. This equates to about 1.5 billion overweight and 500 million obese individuals [3]. Bariatric surgery remains the only evidence-based strategy shown to achieve significant and sustained weight loss in obese individuals [4-6]. Currently, the indications for bariatric surgery in North America include a BMI ≥ 40 kg/m^2 or a BMI ≥ 35 kg/m^2 with obesity-related comorbidities [7,8]. Interestingly, at a recent international consensus, bariatric surgery and specifically laparoscopic sleeve gastrectomy (LSG), was suggested to be indicated for patients with a BMI of 30-35 kg/m^2 with associated obesity-related comorbidities [9]. LSG is a primarily restrictive bariatric procedure that was once the first part of a biliopancreatic diversion with duodenal switch (BPDDS) or a roux-en-Y gastric bypass (RYGB); however recent evidence supports LSG as a standalone procedure [10-15]. Consequently there is increasing research into the effectiveness of LSG as a primary bariatric procedure for obese patients. In this chapter, we will explore LSG as a surgical procedure, focusing on the mechanisms of actions and major outcomes.

Procedure

LSG involves the removal of a large portion of the stomach, leaving a "banana" shaped gastric tube that has significantly reduced capacity (60 to 100mL) [16]. Specifically, patients are positioned in the supine position, following which the greater curvature vessels of the stomach are divided using a harmonic scalpel. The sleeve gastrectomy may be constructed over a 50 French sizing bougie inserted orally, though size of bougie may vary by institution. The antral staple line may be initiated with firings of a linear stapler, followed addition firing as required for the remainder of the stomach. Typically, the staple line is started 4-6 cm proximal to the pylorus. The specimen is usually retrieved with a large endo-pouch. Contrast upper gastrointestinal imaging is performed postoperatively on a selective basis. Typically patients are discharged home on postoperative day 1-3 on a liquid diet. Liquid diets are usually advanced to solid foods slowly. Though sleeve gastrectomy can be performed by the open technique, laparoscopy is less invasive and more commonly chosen. Operating times range from 65-143 minutes, depending on surgeon's experience, training, and institutional setting (i.e. teaching hospital) [11,13,17-21].

One of the benefits of LSG is that it is technically less demanding to perform than some other bariatric surgical procedures such as RYGB. Specifically, there is no gastrointestinal anastomosis, bypass of the duodenum or anastomosis-related complications. Anastomosis-related complications included formation of strictures and the development of leaks [22-25]. Anastomotic strictures result in stenosis of the gastrointestinal lumen and commonly present as with obstructive symptoms in patients. Often treatment of these strictures requires endoscopic dilatation [26,27]. Anastomotic leakage, the most serious complication may lead further operations, and possibly sepsis and death [25,28]. Therefore, with no additional anastomoses during LSG, these significant complications are avoided.

Another advantage of LSG is that it reduces the gastric size without loss of the pyloric sphincter [16]. Specifically, preservation of the pylorus limits dumping syndrome (rapid gastric emptying). Furthermore, no adjustments of bands or devices are needed after the surgery, unlike in adjustable gastric banding. However, disadvantages to the LSG exist. The stomach is stapled during the gastrectomy and there remains a risk gastric leaking or bleeding secondary to compromised staple line integrity [11,29]. As well, LSG is irreversible, unlike adjustable gastric banding. Once the LSG is complete it is virtually impossible to restore the original stomach, which is an important factor that patients need to consider before undergoing the LSG procedure.

Mechanism of Action

LSG is generally defined as a primarily restrictive procedure. By reducing the size of the stomach, the amount of food a person can eat before experiencing a sensation of fullness. Consequently, it was believed that the patient would eat less and weight loss would follow. Additionally, the pyloric sphincter is left intact during LSG, which allows the pyloric sphincter to provide a natural "band effect" that allows the stomach to fill before its contents are released into the small bowel. Though restriction of caloric intake is considered the major component of LSG leading to weight loss, recent research suggests that gastrointestinal hormones changes may play an important role as well.

Satiety is influenced by hormonal signals following filling of the stomach. Ghrelin, is a peptide produced in the fundus of the stomach has been suggested to be a hunger regulating hormone [30-34]. Langer et al. reported significantly reduced plasma levels of the hormone ghrelin following LSG [35]. They suggest that LSG removes most of the ghrelin producing cells and as a result there is a decreased hunger signal. Consequently, patients may decrease intake secondary to both decreased gastric volume and because less ghrelin production signaling satiety. Interestingly, Langer et al. observed that the plasma levels of ghrelin remained low 6 months following LSG [35]. It remains to be determined if ghrelin levels remains decreased in the long-term.

Outcomes

Weight Change

The main objective of LSG is to achieve significant and sustained weight loss in obese individuals. A review by Trelles and Gagner identified 21 studies that involved open and LSG [36]. Overall, based on 1163 patients, the preoperative BMI ranged from 35-74 kg/m^2 and the percent excess weight loss (EWL) at 12 months post-LSG ranged from 45-83%. Based on recent studies, LSG achieves an EWL of 57.7 – 67.5% at one year postoperatively [20,21,37-40]. For instance, a prospective study of 261 patient's by Menenakos et al. reported an EWL of 65.7% at one year following LSG [40].

Interestingly, these authors reported that preoperative BMI > 50 kg/m^2 was predictive of greater weight loss and that weight loss was more rapid in the first 12 months postoperatively. Similar findings have been observed in other studies [20,37-39].

Based on recent studies, decrease in BMI following LSG ranges from 7 – 14.7 kg/m^2 [11,20,21,38,40]. Specifically, we reported in 116 patients (preoperative BMI of 44 kg/m^2) [11] a decrease in BMI of 7 kg/m^2 at one year follow-up post-LSG. In addition, these authors stress the importance of having a comprehensive approach to weight loss, as they observed a

6 kg/m^2 decrease in BMI from lifestyle management alone, in their multidisciplinary obesity clinic prior to surgery.

Common Complications

LSG typically is a low morbidity bariatric surgical procedure. Nevertheless, serious postoperative complications include staple line leakage, bleeding and stricture formation. The management of these complications ranges from conservative to surgical treatment. The overall mortality rate related to LSG is consistently reported as <1% in literature [20,40-42].

Staple line integrity may become compromised resulting in leakage of gastric contents following LSG. Staple line leakage is the most important serious complication, as it may lead to sepsis and death.

A systematic review by Aurora et al, including 29 primary studies and 4888 patients, reported that the leakage rate following LSG is approximately 2.4% [29]. The majority of the leaks occurred at the proximal portion of the gastric staple line., which may be related to the disparate thickness of different sections of the stomach with the fundus being the thinnest [43]. However, many studies did not report the location of the staple line leaks making generalizations difficult [29]. The study by Simon et al which retrospective analyzed 139 patients reported a staple line leakage rate [41] of whom 3.6%. Interestingly, the mean postoperative day of diagnosis of staple line leakage was 13.2 days.

Bleeding from the gastric staple-line is an important complication following LSG. According to Aurora et al., the estimated incidence of bleeding after LSG is 0.7% [29]. In the retrospective studies by Gill et al., Chopra et al., and Simon et al., bleeding rates are reported at 0.9%, 1.1%, and 0%, respectively [11,41,44].

Stricture formation following LSG may lead to stenosis and obstructive symptoms. Aurora et al. estimated the stricture rate following LSG to be 0.5% [29]. However, a retrospective study by Parikh et al reported a 3.5% stricture rate in 230 patients following LSG [45].

These authors suggest that early studies of LSG surgery may underestimate the true incidence of stenosis because larger bougies were used with the intention of LSG being part of a two-stage procedure. Consequently, smaller bougie (ie.36-Fr bougie) may be related to an increased stenosis rate. Similarly, Chopra et al reported a 2.2% obstruction rate following LSG created with a 34-Fr bougie in 185 patients [44]. Conversely, Prasad et al reported no stricture formation in 100 LSG's created with a 36-Fr bougie [20].

Hypertension

Hypertension is a common preoperative obesity-related comorbidity. Based on recent studies the preoperative prevalence of hypertension ranges from 34 - 60% [11,20,39,40,46]. The resolution rate for hypertension following LSG ranges from 42 – 88.8% [20,39,40,46]. Typically, resolution is defined as the ability to cease hypertensive medications and/or achieve a blood pressure lower than 140/90 mmHg. Nonetheless, based on the current evidence, a majority of patients who are hypertensive prior to LSG are likely to experience some improvement in blood pressure following surgery.

Type 2 Diabetes Mellitus

Type 2 diabetes mellitus (T2DM) is another common obesity-related comorbidity. A recent systematic review reported that 66.2% of patients experienced resolution of T2DM following LSG [42]. Resolution, with respect to T2DM, involves cessation of diabetic medication due to improvement in both fasting glucose and HbA1c levels.

Other studies have reported a T2DM resolution rate (after LSG surgery) of 48 – 84% [11,20,39,40,47]. Also, several studies have reported a T2DM improvement rate >80% after LSG surgery [12,17,18,48-52]. However, there is a large amount of heterogeneity in the definition of improvement and in the length of follow-up after surgery.

Prasad et al. reported that 42.7% of 110 patients had T2DM prior to surgery. At 12 months follow-up, 81.2% of the diabetic patients had resolution of their T2DM. In addition, at 36 months follow-up, they reported a 83.3% resolution rate for T2DM [20]. However, only 19% of patients presented for follow-up at 36 months. Consequently, to evaluate long-term success of LSG surgery on both weight and resolution of obesity-related comorbidities, further studies are needed with long-term follow up post-LSG.

Conclusion

In conclusion, LSG has emerged as an effective and safe stand-alone surgery in obese individuals. With LSG producing marked weight loss with low morbidity, it undoubtedly will continue to be an important part of the future of bariatric surgery.

References

[1] Finucane MM, Stevens GA, Cowan MJ, Danaei G, Lin JK, Paciorek CJ, et al. National, regional, and global trends in body-mass index since 1980: systematic analysis of health examination surveys and epidemiological studies with 960 country-years and 9.1 million participants. *Lancet* 2011;377(9765):557-567.

[2] Kelly T, Yang W, Chen CS, Reynolds K, He J. Global burden of obesity in 2005 and projections to 2030. *Int. J. Obes* (Lond) 2008;32(9):1431-1437.

[3] WHO. *Obesity and Overweight.* 2011;Fact sheet 311.

[4] Brethauer SA, Hammel JP, Schauer PR. Systematic review of sleeve gastrectomy as staging and primary bariatric procedure. *Surg. Obes Relat Dis.* 2009;5(4):469-475.

[5] Buchwald H, Avidor Y, Braunwald E, Jensen MD, Pories W, Fahrbach K, et al. Bariatric surgery: a systematic review and meta-analysis. *JAMA* 2004;292(14):1724-1737.

[6] Pontiroli AE, Morabito A. Long-term prevention of mortality in morbid obesity through bariatric surgery. a systematic review and meta-analysis of trials performed with gastric banding and gastric bypass. *Ann. Surg.* 2011;253(3):484-487.

[7] Maggard MA, Shugarman LR, Suttorp M, Maglione M, Sugerman HJ, Livingston EH, et al. Meta-analysis: surgical treatment of obesity. *Ann. Intern. Med.* 2005;142(7): 547-559.

[8] Lau DC, Douketis JD, Morrison KM, Hramiak IM, Sharma AM, Ur E, et al. 2006 Canadian clinical practice guidelines on the management and prevention of obesity in adults and children [summary]. *CMAJ* 2007;176(8):S1-13.

[9] Rosenthal RJ, International Sleeve Gastrectomy Expert Panel, Diaz AA, Arvidsson D, Baker RS, Basso N, et al. International Sleeve Gastrectomy Expert Panel Consensus Statement: best practice guidelines based on experience of >12,000 cases. *Surg. Obes. Relat. Dis*. 2012;8(1):8-19.

[10] Shi X, Karmali S, Sharma AM, Birch DW. A review of laparoscopic sleeve gastrectomy for morbid obesity. *Obes. Surg*. 2010;20(8):1171-1177.

[11] Gill RS, Switzer N, Driedger M, Shi X, Vizhul A, Sharma AM, et al. Laparoscopic Sleeve Gastrectomy with Staple Line Buttress Reinforcement in 116 Consecutive Morbidly Obese Patients. *Obes. Surg*. 2012;22:560-564.

[12] Jacobs M, Bisland W, Gomez E, et al. Laparoscopic sleeve gastrectomy: a retrospective review of 1- and 2-year results. *Surg. Endosc*. 2010;24:781-785.

[13] Braghetto I, Korn O, Valladares H, Gutierrez L, Csendes A, Debandi A, et al. Laparoscopic sleeve gastrectomy: surgical technique, indications and clinical results. *Obes. Surg*. 2007;17(11):1442-1450.

[14] Regan JP, Inabnet WB, Gagner M, Pomp A. Early experience with two-stage laparoscopic Roux-en-Y gastric bypass as an alternative in the super-super obese patient. *Obes. Surg*. 2003;13(6):861-864.

[15] Almogy G, Crookes PF, Anthone GJ. Longitudinal gastrectomy as a treatment for the high-risk super-obese patient. *Obes. Surg* 2004;14(4):492-497.

[16] Frezza EE. Laparoscopic vertical sleeve gastrectomy for morbid obesity. The future procedure of choice? *Surg. Today* 2007;37(4):275-281.

[17] Cottam D, Qureshi FG, Mattar SG, et al. Laparoscopic sleeve gastrectomy as an initial weight-loss procedure for high-risk patients with morbid obesity. *Surg. Endosc*. 2006;20:859-863.

[18] Moon Han S, Kim WW, Oh JH. Results of laparoscopic sleeve gastrectomy (LSG) at 1 year in morbidly obese Korean patients. *Obes. Surg* 2005;15:1469-1475.

[19] Silecchia G, Boru C, Pecchia A, Rizzello M, Casella G, Leonetti F, et al. Effectiveness of laparoscopic sleeve gastrectomy (first stage of biliopancreatic diversion with duodenal switch) on co-morbidities in super-obese high-risk patients. *Obes. Surg*. 2006;16(9):1138-1144.

[20] Prasad P, Tantia O, Patle N, Khanna S, Sen B. An Analysis of 1-3-Year Follow-up Results of Laparoscopic Sleeve Gastrectomy: an Indian Perspective. *Obes. Surg*. 2012;22(3):507-514.

[21] Lee CM, Cirangle PT, Jossart GH. Vertical gastrectomy for morbid obesity in 216 patients: report of two-year results. *Surg. Endosc*. 2007;21(10):1810-1816.

[22] Csendes A, Burgos AM, Burdiles P. Incidence of anastomotic strictures after gastric bypass: a prospective consecutive routine endoscopic study 1 month and 17 months after surgery in 441 patients with morbid obesity. *Obes. Surg*. 2009;19(3):269-273.

[23] Suter M, Donadini A, Calmes JM, Romy S. Improved surgical technique for laparoscopic Roux-en-Y gastric bypass reduces complications at the gastrojejunostomy. *Obes. Surg*. 2010;20(7):841-845.

[24] Ballesta-Lopez C, Poves I, Cabrera M, Almeida JA, Macias G. Learning curve for laparoscopic Roux-en-Y gastric bypass with totally hand-sewn anastomosis: analysis of first 600 consecutive patients. *Surg. Endosc.* 2005;19(4):519-524.

[25] Buckwalter JA, Herbst CA,Jr. Complications of gastric bypass for morbid obesity. *Am. J. Surg*. 1980;139(1):55-60.

[26] Peifer KJ, Shiels AJ, Azar R, Rivera RE, Eagon JC, Jonnalagadda S. Successful endoscopic management of gastrojejunal anastomotic strictures after Roux-en-Y gastric bypass. *Gastrointest Endosc* 2007;66(2):248-252.

[27] Takata MC, Ciovica R, Cello JP, Posselt AM, Rogers SJ, Campos GM. Predictors, treatment, and outcomes of gastrojejunostomy stricture after gastric bypass for morbid obesity. *Obes. Surg*. 2007;17(7):878-884.

[28] Marshall JS, Srivastava A, Gupta SK, Rossi TR, DeBord JR. Roux-en-Y gastric bypass leak complications. *Arch. Surg* 2003;138(5):520-3; discussion 523-4.

[29] Aurora AR, Khaitan L, Saber AA. Sleeve gastrectomy and the risk of leak: a systematic analysis of 4,888 patients. Surg Endosc 2011 Dec 17.

[30] Kojima M, Hosoda H, Date Y, Nakazato M, Matsuo H, Kangawa K. Ghrelin is a growth-hormone-releasing acylated peptide from stomach. Nature 1999;402(6762): 656-660.

[31] Ariyasu H, Takaya K, Tagami T, Ogawa Y, Hosoda K, Akamizu T, et al. Stomach is a major source of circulating ghrelin, and feeding state determines plasma ghrelin-like immunoreactivity levels in humans. *J. Clin. Endocrinol. Metab* 2001;86(10):4753-4758.

[32] Gnanapavan S, Kola B, Bustin SA, Morris DG, McGee P, Fairclough P, et al. The tissue distribution of the mRNA of ghrelin and subtypes of its receptor, GHS-R, in humans. *J. Clin. Endocrinol. Metab.* 2002;87(6):2988.

[33] Wren AM, Small CJ, Ward HL, Murphy KG, Dakin CL, Taheri S, et al. The novel hypothalamic peptide ghrelin stimulates food intake and growth hormone secretion. *Endocrinology* 2000;141(11):4325-4328.

[34] Wren AM, Seal LJ, Cohen MA, Brynes AE, Frost GS, Murphy KG, et al. Ghrelin enhances appetite and increases food intake in humans. *J. Clin. Endocrinol. Metab.* 2001;86(12):5992.

[35] Langer FB, Reza Hoda MA, Bohdjalian A, Felberbauer FX, Zacherl J, Wenzl E, et al. Sleeve gastrectomy and gastric banding: effects on plasma ghrelin levels. *Obes. Surg* 2005;15(7):1024-1029.

[36] Trelles N, Gagner M. Updated review of sleeve gastrectomy. *Open Gastroentero J.* 2008;2:41-49.

[37] Himpens J, Dapri G, Cadiere GB. A prospective randomized study between laparoscopic gastric banding and laparoscopic isolated sleeve gastrectomy: results after 1 and 3 years. *Obes. Surg*. 2006;16(11):1450-1456.

[38] Arias E, Martinez PR, Ka Ming Li V, Szomstein S, Rosenthal RJ. Mid-term follow-up after sleeve gastrectomy as a final approach for morbid obesity. *Obes. Surg.* 2009;19(5):544-548.

[39] Sammour T, Hill AG, Singh P, Ranasinghe A, Babor R, Rahman H. Laparoscopic sleeve gastrectomy as a single-stage bariatric procedure. *Obes. Surg*. 2010;20(3):271-275.

[40] Menenakos E, Stamou KM, Albanopoulos K, Papailiou J, Theodorou D, Leandros E. Laparoscopic sleeve gastrectomy performed with intent to treat morbid obesity: a prospective single-center study of 261 patients with a median follow-up of 1 year. *Obes. Surg.* 2010;20(3):276-282.

[41] Simon TE, Scott JA, Brockmeyer JR, Rice RC, Frizzi JD, Husain FA, et al. Comparison of staple-line leakage and hemorrhage in patients undergoing laparoscopic sleeve gastrectomy with or without seamguard. *Am. Surg.* 2011;77(12):1665-1668.

[42] Gill RS, Birch DW, Shi X, Sharma AM, Karmali S. Sleeve gastrectomy and type 2 diabetes mellitus: a systematic review. *Surg. Obes. Relat Dis* 2010;6(6):707-713.

[43] Elariny H, Gonzalez H, Wang B. Tissue thickness of human stomach measured on excised gastric specimens from obese patients. *Surg. Technol. Int.* 2005;14:119-124.

[44] Chopra A, Chao E, Etkin Y, Merklinger L, Lieb J, Delany H. Laparoscopic sleeve gastrectomy for obesity: can it be considered a definitive procedure? *Surg. Endosc.* 2012;26(3):831-837.

[45] Parikh A, Alley JB, Peterson RM, Harnisch MC, Pfluke JM, Tapper DM, et al. Management options for symptomatic stenosis after laparoscopic vertical sleeve gastrectomy in the morbidly obese. *Surg. Endosc.* 2012;26(3):738-746.

[46] Weiner RA, Weiner S, Pomhoff I, Jacobi C, Makarewicz W, Weigand G. Laparoscopic sleeve gastrectomy--influence of sleeve size and resected gastric volume. *Obes. Surg.* 2007;17(10):1297-1305.

[47] Abbatini F, Rizzello M, Casella G, Alessandri G, Capoccia D, Leonetti F, et al. Long-term effects of laparoscopic sleeve gastrectomy, gastric bypass, and adjustable gastric banding on type 2 diabetes. *Surg. Endosc* 2010;24(5):1005-1010.

[48] Lakdawala MA, Bhasker A, Mulchandani D, Goel S, Jain S. Comparison between the results of laparoscopic sleeve gastrectomy and laparoscopic Roux-en-Y gastric bypass in the Indian population: a retrospective 1 year study. *Obes. Surg.* 2010;6:707-713.

[49] Lirosi F, El Kallaawi M, Batterham RL, Adamo M. Do we need bypass surgery to cure diabetes? Prompt remission of diabetes after laparoscopic sleeve gastrectomy - a UK experience. *Surg. Obes. Relat Dis.* 2010;6:229-230.

[50] Shah S, Todkar J, Shah P. Effect of laparoscopic sleeve gastrectomy (LSG) on HbA1c levels in T2DM patients: results after one year. Obes Surg IFSO 2009;Abstract P-071.

[51] Chowbey PK, Dhawan K, Khullar R, et al. Laparoscopic sleeve gastrectomy: an Indian experience - surgical technique and early results. *Obes. Surg.* 2010;20:1340-1347.

[52] Vidal J, Ibarzabal A, Romero F, et al. Type 2 diabetes mellitus and the metabolic syndrome following sleeve gastrectomy in severely obese subjects. *Obes. Surg.* 2008;18:1077-1082.

In: The Fundamentals of Bariatric Surgery
Editors: Shahzeer Karmali and Daniel W. Birch
ISBN: 978-1-62417-732-3

Chapter 11

The Role of Laparoscopy in Bariatric Surgery: The Shift from Open to Laparoscopic Approaches

Ashley Vergis and Krista Hardy
Department of Surgery, University of Manitoba,
Winnipeg, Canada

Abstract

Irrespective of a laparoscopic or open technique, the objectives of bariatric surgery endure. Namely, they are to extend and improve quality of life, obviate weight-related comorbidities, and to realize and sustain meaningful weight loss. Furthermore, these objectives must be achieved in an efficacious and cost-effective manner. The history of obesity surgery is storied. There has been considerable evolution, and indeed extinction, in the procedures performed. This chapter will review open and laparocopic surgery in the obese patient, bariatric surgery pre laparoscopy, the conventional laparoscopic bariatric surgery and finally the way forward including single incision bariatric surgery.

Open vs. Laparoscopic Surgery in the Obese Patient

It is well established that the overall risk of morbidity and mortality for a given individual increases with the degree of their obesity (Stevens, Cai et al. 1998; Calle, Thun et al. 1999). A synopsis of this issue is beyond the scope of this chapter and can be found elsewhere in this textbook and in other general readings. What is of relevance is the negative synergistic effect that obesity and the laparotomy incision have on bariatric patients and their surgeons.

From the patient's perspective, increased adiposity fosters a pro-inflammatory milieu due to a host of mediators including increased levels of factors such as C-reactive protein, interleukin 1β, tumour necrosis factor α, and transforming growth factor β, amongst others.

This pro-inflammatory state is associated with obesity-related comorbidities that place bariatric patients at increased perioperative risk(Cottam, Nguyen et al. 2005). These include obesity hypoventilation syndrome, type II diabetes, sleep apnea, and artheriosclerotic disease. Regardless of open or laparoscopic technique, careful preoperative optimization of these comorbidities is imperative for satisfactory outcomes.

The relevant primary differences between open and laparoscopic approaches can be viewed as the positive effects of reduced tissue injury and the negative effects of the carbon dioxide (CO2) pneumoperitoneum in laparoscopy.

Tissue Injury and Pulmonary Function

The degree of surgical injury will determine the host's biological response while the host's underlying capacity will determine its overall ability to recover. As outlined, bariatric surgical patients are often burdened with conditions that test their physiologic reserve.

One goal of laparoscopy is to minimize this maladaptive response by substantially reducing tissue injury to the patient while affecting the same surgical outcome. Laparoscopy provides a means of limiting injury and reducing the stress response by providing superior view and access to target organs, eliminating large upper-midline incisions, reducing visceral manipulation, and minimizing body wall retraction. These factors have been shown to reduce fluid third-space fluid loss, substantially decrease perioperative intra-abdominal pressure, and attenuate the response of pro-inflammatory mediators. The pulmonary benefit is also apparent.

Those undergoing laparoscopy tend to have less pain and associated chest wall splinting, tachypnea, and postoperative atelectasis. Objectively, this can be seen in laparoscopic cohorts using less analgesia, requiring less supplemental oxygen and having improved pulmonary function parameters such forced vital capacity, forced expiratory volume (1 sec and mid expiratory), and peak expiratory flows, compared to their open counterparts (Schauer, Luna et al. 1993).

Thromboembolic Complications

Virchow's triad of endothelial injury, venous stasis, and hypercoaguabilty illustrate the thromboembolic perils morbidly obese patients face when undergoing any intervention. Although the laparoscopic approach does lower thromboembolic risks in some regards (decreased tissue injury, decreased inflammatory/pro-coagulative mediators, earlier ambulation), it amplifies others.

A significant factor related to venous thromboembolism is the CO2 pneumoperitoneum. The increased intra-abdominal pressure decreases venous return and flow in the lower extremities thus promoting venous stasis (Nguyen, Cronan et al. 2003).

Patient positioning is also a factor. Surgeons often employ extreme reverse trendelenberg to gain sufficient access and view. This further promotes venous pooling and stasis . Finally, operative times may be prolonged with surgeons who are early in their learning curve.

This compounds the aforementioned concerns. As such, those employing laparoscopic techniques in their bariatric practice are encouraged to use minimal insufflation pressures and judicious bed positioning in order to obtain adequate and safe visualization.

These guidelines along with the use of preoperative subcutaneous anticoagulants and intermittent sequential lower extremity compression devices will reduce the risk of thromboembolic complications to less than 1% in those undergoing laparoscopic bariatric procedures as compared to approximately 3% in open groups.

Bariatric Surgery - The Pre Laparoscopic Era

Bariatric surgery debuted in the 1950's with intestinal bypass procedures that utilized malabsorption to treat severe hyperlipidemia. Bariatric surgery was perhaps made infamous with introduction of the ileo-jejunal bypass of the mid 1970's. Although there are several variants, essentially, the proximal jejunum is anastomosed to the distal ileum with the majority of the small bowel's absorptive capacity being bypassed. The excluded segment was either left blind or anastomosed to other hollow viscera such as the colon, stomach or even the biliary tract. Although lipid and weight control were excellent, patients developed other significant side effects including incapacitating steatorrhea, nutritional deficiencies, oxalate stones, arthropathy, and a 2% incidence of liver failure (DeWind and Payne 1976; Zollinger, Coccia et al. 1983). Currently most bariatric procedures are restrictive in nature based on this record. The malabsorptive operations including biliopancreatic diversion (BPD) and its modification, BPD with duodenal switch (DS), account for less than 5% of bariatric surgical procedures performed (Buchwald and Williams 2004). Surgeons performing these malabsorptive procedures must understand their potential for metabolic and nutritional derangements.

Gastric bypass was first described in the 1960's by Mason and Itoh (EE and C 1969). As a primarily restrictive operation with a minor malabsorptive component, the procedure generally involved isolating a restrictive gastric pouch and anastomosing it to a bypassed segment of small bowel of variable length. Later, it was widely popularized with the Roux-en-Y (RYGB) modification making it the relative gold standard throughout the 1990's (Griffen, Young et al. 1977; Schirmer 2006).

The 1980's brought forth a new generation of restrictive bariatric surgery including procedures such as the vertical banded gastroplasty (VBG). In this procedure, a circular window was created in the stomach below and to the patient's left of the gastroesophageal junction. A vertical non-cutting staple line was then placed from the window cephalad to create a small pouch. Restriction was then achieved by placing a non-adjustable polyurethane band around the bottom of the pouch through the circular window and around the lesser curvature of the stomach (Mason 1982).

The VBG enjoyed initial widespread application due to its technical ease and early favorable results. Unfortunately, this success was short lived when follow up revealed significant patient intolerance of high fiber diets. This often led to patients ingesting high calorie liquids that reduced the procedure's long-term efficacy (Brolin, Robertson et al. 1994). The dietary issues, coupled with the difficulty of reversing or revising the procedure due to excessive scarring around the band in the case of complications, have largely led to abandonment of the VBG.

Bariatric Surgery- The Laparoscopic Era

Interestingly, obesity was generally viewed as a contraindication during the early period of laparoscopic surgery. With increasing experience and technologic advances, laparoscopy has now been applied to almost all intra-abdominal procedures. Indeed, the majority of bariatric operations are now performed using the laparoscope.

A new era in bariatric surgery unfolded with the placement of the first nonadjustable gastric band by Catona in Italy in 1992 (Catona, Gossenberg et al. 1993). The laparoscopic adjustable gastric band (LAGB) then placed by Belachew in 1993, further popularized this form of bariatric surgery largely due to its technical simplicity and low perioperative complication rate (Belachew, Legrand et al. 2001). However, the early perigastric technique of band insertion was associated with a high degree of band complications including slippage and erosion.

This prompted a transition to the current pars flaccida technique. After gaining popularity in Australia and Europe, the LAGB was approved by the FDA in the United States and Health Canada. This greatly increased the number of bands placed globally. Currently, the LAGB is one of the most popular bariatric procedures worldwide.

Wittgrove, Clark and Tremblay performed the first laparoscopic RYGB in 1993 (Wittgrove, Clark et al. 1994). This was considered a formidable accomplishment due to the technical challenges of this procedure. The technique employed a retrocolic retrogastric roux limb and a circular stapled gastrojejunostomy. Experience grew with the LRYGB over the following years and several randomized trials were performed that confirmed the benefits of the laparoscopic approach (Nguyen, Goldman et al. 2001; Westling and Gustavsson 2001). These include reduced wound complications, incisional hernias, postoperative pain, respiratory complications and length of stay.

There are certain variations on technique including the approach for anastamosis (circular stapler, linear stapler, hand-sewn, robot-assisted) and roux limb (antecolic, antegastric). With experience, the morbidity and mortality associated with LRYGB has reduced significantly with the operative time now less than two hours, length of stay often less than 24h and mortality rates less than 0.5% (Schauer, Ikramuddin et al. 2003; McCarty, Arnold et al. 2005; Shikora, Kim et al. 2005; Flum, Belle et al. 2009).

The laparoscopic approach has also been applied to the most complex bariatric procedures, including BPD and DS. These procedures have the greatest magnitude of weight loss but are associated with increased postoperative morbidity including significant nutritional deficiencies. Few surgeons perform these procedures regularly. Ren, Patterson and Gagner described a laparoscopic DS procedure in 1999 (Ren, Patterson et al. 2000). This was associated with a relatively high mortality rate that prompted the introduction of a two-stage operation with laparoscopic sleeve gastrectomy (LSG) as the initial procedure. Further experience has improved the safety of the laparoscopic approach but it still remains a relatively uncommon procedure.

After introduction of LSG in the staged DS, this procedure was also employed by other centers as a primary weight loss procedure for high-risk patients and the super-obese (BMI>60) (Baltasar, Serra et al. 2005). With a significant proportion of patients having an acceptable primary result and forgoing the second stage procedure, LSG is now offered as a single procedure for patients in the lower BMI categories with satisfactory intermediate outcomes. Longer-term outcomes in terms of weight loss and comorbidity resolution are still unknown.

Single Incision Laparoscopic Surgery

In recent years, the field of laparoscopy has evolved rapidly with new advances in single incision laparoscopic surgery (SILS). SILS is a technique that employs a single multi-access port along with conventional laparoscopic instruments. At present, experience with SILS bariatrics is limited to small case series by surgeons with significant experience in this novel technique. While there are obvious cosmetic advantages to a single incision, the long-term outcomes of SILS bariatric surgery are yet unknown.

SILS was initially described for adjustable gastric banding and sleeve gastrectomy in 2008 (Nguyen, Hinojosa et al. 2008; Saber, Elgamal et al. 2008). These procedures are considered to be less technically demanding than other bariatric operations and already require extension of a port incision for band insertion or specimen extraction. This extended incision was initially considered a natural site for SILS port access. However, the technique was subsequently modified to employ an umbilical incision for improved cosmesis. A small study on SILS sleeve gastrectomy demonstrated less postoperative pain, lower need for analgesia and decreased length of hospital stay compared to conventional multi-port laparoscopic sleeve gastrectomy (Saber, El-Ghazaly et al. 2010).

More recently SILS has been applied to gastric bypass and biliopancreatic diversion (Huang, Yao et al. 2010; Tacchino, Greco et al. 2010).

Some experts perform a single loop gastric bypass procedure with one anastamosis to simplify the technical aspects but a double loop Roux-en-Y technique has also been described.

Obese patients present their own unique challenges because of liver bulk and extensive intra-abdominal adipose tissue. Traditional multi-port bariatric surgery typically employs a Nathanson retractor to elevate the left lateral segment of the liver. Various liver retraction techniques have been developed with SILS in order to avoid the incision required for Nathanson insertion including transfixation sutures, liver-puncturing suspension tapes, penrose drains and retraction using the elevated stomach (de la Torre, Satgunam et al. 2009; Huang, Houng et al. 2009; Tacchino, Greco et al. 2010; Huang, Lo et al. 2011).

SILS bariatric surgery is currently limited to high volume surgeons with significant SILS experience. There are potential advances on the horizon in the areas of semi-flexible endoscopy and instrument triangulation that will likely facilitate the procedure in larger patients. Long-term results including the risk of incisional hernia are still unknown and further well-designed randomized trials are required to assess these outcomes. Nonetheless, SILS bariatric surgery is a technically feasible and safe procedure when performed by an experienced surgeon on well-selected patients.

References

Baltasar, A., C. Serra, et al. (2005). "Laparoscopic sleeve gastrectomy: a multi-purpose bariatric operation." *Obes. Surg.* 15(8): 1124-1128.

Belachew, M., M. J. Legrand, et al. (2001). "History of Lap-Band: from dream to reality." *Obes. Surg.* 11(3): 297-302.

Brolin, R. L., L. B. Robertson, et al. (1994). "Weight loss and dietary intake after vertical banded gastroplasty and Roux-en-Y gastric bypass." *Ann. Surg.* 220(6): 782-790.

Buchwald, H. and S. E. Williams (2004). "Bariatric surgery worldwide 2003." Obes Surg 14(9): 1157-1164.

Calle, E. E., M. J. Thun, et al. (1999). "Body-mass index and mortality in a prospective cohort of U.S. adults." *N. Engl J. Med.* 341(15): 1097-1105.

Catona, A., M. Gossenberg, et al. (1993). "Laparoscopic Gastric Banding: preliminary series." *Obes. Surg.* 3(2): 207-209.

Cottam, D. R., N. T. Nguyen, et al. (2005). "The impact of laparoscopy on bariatric surgery." *Surg. Endosc.* 19(5): 621-627.

de la Torre, R. A., S. Satgunam, et al. (2009). "Transumbilical single-port laparoscopic adjustable gastric band placement with liver suture retractor." *Obes. Surg.* 19(12): 1707-1710.

DeWind, L. T. and J. H. Payne (1976). "Intestinal bypass surgery for morbid obesity. Long-term results." *JAMA* 236(20): 2298-2301.

EE, M. and I. C (1969). "Gastric bypass in obesity." *Surg. Clin. North Am.* 47: 1345-1351.

Flum, D. R., S. H. Belle, et al. (2009). "Perioperative safety in the longitudinal assessment of bariatric surgery." *N. Engl. J. Med.* 361(5): 445-454.

Griffen, W. O., Jr., V. L. Young, et al. (1977). "A prospective comparison of gastric and jejunoileal bypass procedures for morbid obesity." *Ann. Surg.* 186(4): 500-509.

Huang, C. K., J. Y. Houng, et al. (2009). "Single incision transumbilical laparoscopic Roux-en-Y gastric bypass: a first case report." *Obes. Surg.* 19(12): 1711-1715.

Huang, C. K., C. H. Lo, et al. (2011). "A novel technique for liver retraction in laparoscopic bariatric surgery." *Obes. Surg.* 21(5): 676-679.

Huang, C. K., S. F. Yao, et al. (2010). "A novel surgical technique: single-incision transumbilical laparoscopic Roux-en-Y gastric bypass." *Obes. Surg.* 20(10): 1429-1435.

Mason, E. E. (1982). "Vertical banded gastroplasty for obesity." *Arch. Surg.* 117(5): 701-706.

McCarty, T. M., D. T. Arnold, et al. (2005). "Optimizing outcomes in bariatric surgery: outpatient laparoscopic gastric bypass." *Ann. Surg.* 242(4): 494-498; discussion 498-501.

Nguyen, N. T., M. Cronan, et al. (2003). "Duplex ultrasound assessment of femoral venous flow during laparoscopic and open gastric bypass." *Surg. Endosc.* 17(2): 285-290.

Nguyen, N. T., C. Goldman, et al. (2001). "Laparoscopic versus open gastric bypass: a randomized study of outcomes, quality of life, and costs." *Ann. Surg.* 234(3): 279-289; discussion 289-291.

Nguyen, N. T., M. W. Hinojosa, et al. (2008). "Single laparoscopic incision transabdominal (SLIT) surgery-adjustable gastric banding: a novel minimally invasive surgical approach." *Obes. Surg.* 18(12): 1628-1631.

Ren, C. J., E. Patterson, et al. (2000). "Early results of laparoscopic biliopancreatic diversion with duodenal switch: a case series of 40 consecutive patients." *Obes. Surg.* 10(6): 514-523; discussion 524.

Saber, A. A., T. H. El-Ghazaly, et al. (2010). "Single-incision laparoscopic sleeve gastrectomy versus conventional multiport laparoscopic sleeve gastrectomy: technical considerations and strategic modifications." *Surg. Obes Relat Dis.* 6(6): 658-664.

Saber, A. A., M. H. Elgamal, et al. (2008). "Single incision laparoscopic sleeve gastrectomy (SILS): a novel technique." *Obes. Surg.* 18(10): 1338-1342.

Schauer, P., S. Ikramuddin, et al. (2003). "The learning curve for laparoscopic Roux-en-Y gastric bypass is 100 cases." *Surg. Endosc.* 17(2): 212-215.

Schauer, P. R., J. Luna, et al. (1993). "Pulmonary function after laparoscopic cholecystectomy." *Surgery* 114(2): 389-397; discussion 397-389.

Schirmer, B. (2006). "Laparoscopic bariatric surgery." *Surg. Endosc.* 20 Suppl 2: S450-455.

Shikora, S. A., J. J. Kim, et al. (2005). "Laparoscopic Roux-en-Y gastric bypass: results and learning curve of a high-volume academic program." *Arch. Surg.* 140(4): 362-367.

Stevens, J., J. Cai, et al. (1998). "The effect of age on the association between body-mass index and mortality." *N. Engl. J. Med.* 338(1): 1-7.

Tacchino, R. M., F. Greco, et al. (2010). "Laparoscopic gastric banding without visible scar: a short series with intraumbilical SILS." *Obes. Surg.* 20(2): 236-239.

Tacchino, R. M., F. Greco, et al. (2010). "Single-incision laparoscopic gastric bypass for morbid obesity." *Obes. Surg.* 20(8): 1154-1160.

Westling, A. and S. Gustavsson (2001). "Laparoscopic vs open Roux-en-Y gastric bypass: a prospective, randomized trial." *Obes. Surg.* 11(3): 284-292.

Wittgrove, A. C., G. W. Clark, et al. (1994). "Laparoscopic Gastric Bypass, Roux-en-Y: Preliminary Report of Five Cases." *Obes. Surg.* 4(4): 353-357.

Zollinger, R. W., M. R. Coccia, et al. (1983). "Critical analysis of jejunoileal bypass." *Am. J. Surg.* 146(5): 626-630.

In: The Fundamentals of Bariatric Surgery
Editors: Shahzeer Karmali and Daniel W. Birch

ISBN: 978-1-62417-732-3

Chapter 12

Emerging Techniques in Bariatric Surgery

Kourosh Sarkhosh[1], Niroshan Sothilingam[1], Noah Switzer[1] and Shahzeer Karmali[1,2,*]

[1]Center for the Advancement of Minimally Invasive Surgery (CAMIS), Royal Alexandra Hospital, Edmonton, Alberta, Canada
[2]Department of Surgery, University of Alberta, Edmonton, Canada

Abstract

Obesity is a major health problem worldwide affecting both adults and children and is the second most common preventable cause of mortality in North America. To quantify this issue, more than 30% of the population in North America can be classified as obese. Bariatric surgery is currently the only modality that results in a sustained longterm weight loss, along with resolution of obesity-related comorbidities, like diabetes. However, these procedures are not without consequences, as they can be associated with significant morbidity and mortality. In an effort to reduce the complications associated with bariatric surgical procedures, alternative endoscopic and endoluminal techniques have been developed. In this chapter, these emerging techniques will be reviewed.

Introduction

Obesity is a major health problem worldwide and is the second most common preventable cause of death in North America. [1] It is responsible for a multitude of medical comorbidities, it has been strongly associated with an increased incidence of diabetes,

* Corresponding author: Dr. Shahzeer Karmali, Center for the Advancement of Minimally Invasive Surgery (CAMIS), Royal Alexandra Hospital, 10240 Kingsway, Edmonton, Alberta, T5H 3V9, Canada. Phone: (780) 735-6650; Fax: (780) 735-6652. E-mail: shahzeer@ualberta.ca.

cardiovascular disease and cancer. [2, 3] Although diet and exercise programs are considered the pillars for the treatment of obesity, long-term studies have failed to show a sustained weight loss for the vast majority of these patients. [2]

Currently, bariatric surgery is the only modality that results in a sustained weight loss along with reversal of obesity-related comorbidities. [4] Excess weight loss (EWL) in patients with morbid obesity reaches 47.5 –70.1% following bariatic surgery. [5]

Since the introduction of laparoscopic surgery in 1987 by Mouret, an increasing amount of surgeons are utilizing this method for the treatment of various diseases. [6] In the field of bariatric surgery, procedures such as Roux-en-Y gastric bypass (RYGB), sleeve gastrectomy and adjustable gastric banding are frequently performed laparoscopically. However, complications associated with these procedures such as infection, bleeding, anastomotic leak or stricture, incisional hernia, fistula or mortality affect a considerable number of patients post-operatively.

Furthermore, there still remains a large mismatch between the number of patients requiring these procedures and those who actually receive it. Therefore, there has been a push amongst surgeons and investigators towards introducing a less invasive and more readily-available procedure for the treatment of morbid obesity. More specifically, flexible endoscopy has become an invaluable tool used in treatment of patients with morbid obesity.

Intragastric Balloons

Intragastric balloons (IGBs) are one of the older devices used for the treatment of obesity. [7] Their initial use was associated with a disappointing high number of complications such as bowel obstruction. Newer devices have since been developed with slightly better outcomes.

The balloon is deployed in the stomach under direct vision using endoscopy and inflated with roughly 500-700 cc of saline or methylene blue solution. Importantly, removal of the device is easy as the operator can deflate the balloon using a variety of needles or endoscopic snares.

In a retrospective analysis, Genco et al. reported an EWL of 33% +/- 18.7% at 6 months follow-up after placement of IGB's. Improvement or resolution of diabetes and hypertension was observed in 86.9% and 93.7% of patients, respectively. [8]

However, two thirds of their patients developed severe nausea and vomiting which lead to early removal of some balloons. Other complications included early accidental deflation of the balloon and gastric ulceration or erosion. [9, 10]

These authors reported an overall complication rate of 2.8%. This included 5 patients who developed gastric perforation, 2 of whom subsequently died. [8] In another longer meta-analysis, Ercan et al. recorded results after 5 years of follow-up. [11]

These investigators reported a weight loss of $\geq$ 10% in less than a third of their patients. The long-term data for weight loss associated with IGB's is unfortunately not currently available.

Endoluminal Vertical Gastroplasty

Initially developed for the treatment of gastroesophageal reflux disease (GERD), the endoluminal vertical gastroplasty (EndoCinch) is a suturing device contained within a capsule, attached to a gastroscope. [9] Plication of the gastroesophageal junction (GEJ) is perfomed with this device, with the intent of improving or resolving the patient's GERD. However, with the lack of significant results showing longterm resolution of GERD, it was found to be futile in this manner. [9, 12] Interestingly, with these sutures in place, distention of the stomach was severely limited. Fogel et al. took advantage of this fact and first described the use of the EndoCinch for the treatment of morbid obesity. [13] They reported EWL values at 21.1% and 58.1% at 1 and 12 months, respectively. Fourteen patients underwent a repeat endoscopy during their follow-up to assess their suture line. Of these, 5 had intact suture lines, 6 patients had relatively intact suture lines, but not as intact as the day of the procedure, and 3 patients had disruption of their suture line requiring further intervention. [13]

Transoral Gastroplasty

This is an endoscopic stapling system which creates a full thickness plication of the proximal stomach. [9, 14] A prospective European study by Familiari et al. investigated the safety and efficacy of transoral gastroplasty (TOGA) in a multicentered trial. [15] These investigators described the procedure by starting with a diagnostic gastroscopy. A stiff guidewire is then placed into the stomach and bougie dialators are subsequently used to stretch the esophagous and asssess its resistance. The stapler is then introduced over the guidewire into the proximal stomach. A small caliber gastroscope is advanced through the device and retroflexed to directly visualize the stapler. Next, starting at the level of the GE junction, using vacuum pods with suction, the anterior and posterior stomach walls are drawn into the stapler. The stapler is closed and fired, allowing serosa-to-serosa apposition parallel to the lesser curvature of the stomach creating a gastric sleeve. The stapler is then removed, reloaded and the procedure is repeated for the total length of approximately 8 cm. Patients get discharged the following day following a contrast swallow study to rule out any leaks. Solid food was introduced on average at 4 weeks post-operatively. [14]

Data is available in 53 of their 67 studied patients at 1 year followup. The EWL was at 29.3% +/- 11.6%, 36.8% +/- 15.7%, and 38.7% +/- 17.1% at 3, 6, and 12 months, respectively. Hemoglobin A1C levels decreased from 5.9% at baseline to 5.4% at 12 months for all patients (P<.001). Triglyceride (TG) levels were significantly decreased from 142.9 mg/dL at baseline to 98.0 mg/dL at 12 months (P<.0001). High-density lipoprotein (HDL) levels significantly increased from 47.0 mg/dL at baseline to 57.5 mg/dL at 12 months (P<.0001). In contrast, patients' blood pressure was not significantly improved at 12 months. It was also reported that almost half of the patients had a small dehiscence of the staple line, discovered on follow-up endoscopy. [14] These authors concluded that TOGA can produce similar outcomes to other restrictive bariatric procedures such as gastric banding or endoluminal vertical gastroplasty. [9, 14] The potential limitations to this study included a short follow-up time of 1 year and the small sample size (n = 67 patients), as well as significant loss to follow-up, with 21% of patients lost within that first year.

Endoluminal Sleeve

One of the first true endoluminal devices used to bypass the proximal small intestine is the duodenojejunal bypass sleeve. This is a self-expanding implant that is placed in the duodenum and attached to a plastic sleeve that extends into the proximal jejunum. The device is usually preloaded onto a wire-guided catheter system that is advanced into the small bowel under fluoroscopy. Rodriguez-Grunert et al. described the procedure as deploying the sleeve by pushing the inner sheath of the catheter into the proximal jejunum. [16] Once the sleeve is fully extended, a self-expanding anchor is released in the duodenal bulb to hold the device in place.

In animal studies, weight loss and improved glucose metabolism was observed by Agruirre et al., when comparing RYGB with a nutrient-impermeable endoluminal sleeve (ELS). [2] This flexible tube is designed to be positioned at the duodenal bulb and extend into the proximal jejunum. It will cause ingested food to bypass directly into the jejunum. The mucosa of the proximal jejunum is therefore exposed to nutrients that has not been affected by pancreaticobiliary secretions or digestive functions of the proximal gut. These investiagtors concluded that ELS mimics many of the effects of RYGB in their rat model. Although ELS induces only about two-thirds as much weight loss as RYGB in the same strain of rats, the effect on glucose homeostasis is comparable to that observed after RYGB. [2] While gastric emptying was not formally measured, the study mentions that using fluoroscopic assessment seemed to be slowed after ELS implantation. The substantial effect of ELS on glucose homeostasis compared to weight loss suggests an important role for the duodenum and jejunum in the regulation of this metabolic function. Fasting ghrelin levels were unchanged after ELS-induced weight loss, a result also found with RYBG. [17] Ghrelin, is a potent peripherally active orexigenic hormone found in the gastric fundus, thought to be responsible for the hunger drive. [2] It is the suppression of this hormone that allows weight loss.

Sandler et al. compared ELS technique to mimic the restrictive and malabsorptive features of the RYGB in a short, prospective, single-center human trial. [18] A gastroduodenojejunal bypass sleeve was anchored at the gastroesophageal junction and acted as a endoluminal gastroduodenojejunal bypass. Seventeen patients maintained the device for the 12 week duration of the study. The trial was designed to show the short-term follow-up and safety of the gastroduodenojejunal bypass. An average of 39.7% EWL was observed at the 12 week follow-up. Out of these 17 patients, 12 had previous comorbidities, including diabetes mellitus type 2, hypertension, and hyperlipidemia. With the implantation of the device, all diabetic patients no longer required medications to control their disease. Patients were able to stop their antihypertensive medications. Those with hyperlipidema had seen a normalization of their levels by the end of the study. [18] The device, therefore, functioned with both a malabsorptive mechanism, limiting nutritional absorption, and a restrictive one, limiting food intake. Adverse effects such as dehydration, diarrhea, abdominal pain were not seen in the group that finished the trial in the short-term. In the early device development, laparoscopic visualization was used to ensure that the suture attachment of the device to the GE junction was full thickness. The authors postulate that with practice and improvements, this step can be eliminated, making this procedure completely endoluminal in nature. [18]

Conclusion

With an increasing demand for less-invasive procedures for the surgical management of various diseases, the use of incisionless bariatric surgical interventions will likely rise in the near future. In order for these techniques to become popular, not only should they cause a meaningful and sustained decrease in BMI, they should also diminish the comorbidities associated with obesity. However, the use of endoluminal techniques for the treatment of obesity is presently still in its early state. Not only is the amount of human data being quite limited, but the acquisition of such data is challenging, as it is difficult to design human studies for weight loss devices. This is due to the fact there are numerous confounding variables, strong placebo effects and unique patient experiences to diet and exercise regimens. The ideal design would require a randomized, controlled, double-blinded study with identical dietary, exercise and educational controls. To the best of our knoweldge, there has not been a study that we have reviewed that has been conducted in this manner.

There is however substantial evidence in the literature suggesting the durability and effectiveness of current weight loss procedures such as RYGB. To date, no endoluminal technique can reproduce the substantial weight loss and metabolic effects of the RYGB. The available literature for endoluminal procedures has only shown short-term success. The belief is that an endoluminal approach potentially can be a safer alternative and could offer an intervention to those with obesity and its related illnesses. If endoluminal technology is to be strongly considered as a primary weight loss procedure then definitive outcome measures, as well as design and execution for a prospective, randomized, double-blind trial must be studied.

References

[1] Flegal, K.M., et al., Prevalence and trends in obesity among US adults, 1999-2008. *JAMA*, 2010. 303(3): p. 235-41.

[2] Aguirre, V., et al., An endoluminal sleeve induces substantial weight loss and normalizes glucose homeostasis in rats with diet-induced obesity. *Obesity* (Silver Spring), 2008. 16(12): p. 2585-92.

[3] Whitlock, G., et al., Body-mass index and cause-specific mortality in 900 000 adults: collaborative analyses of 57 prospective studies. *Lancet*, 2009. 373(9669): p. 1083-96.

[4] Sjostrom, L., et al., Effects of bariatric surgery on mortality in Swedish obese subjects. *N. Engl. J. Med.,* 2007. 357(8): p. 741-52.

[5] Buchwald, H., et al., Bariatric surgery: a systematic review and meta-analysis. *JAMA*, 2004. 292(14): p. 1724-37.

[6] Spaner, S.J. and G.L. Warnock, A brief history of endoscopy, laparoscopy, and laparoscopic surgery. *J. Laparoendosc. Adv. Surg. Tech. A*, 1997. 7(6): p. 369-73.

[7] Hogan, R.B., et al., A double-blind, randomized, sham-controlled trial of the gastric bubble for obesity. *Gastrointest. Endosc.*, 1989. 35(5): p. 381-5.
[8] Genco, A., et al., BioEnterics Intragastric Balloon: The Italian Experience with 2,515 Patients. *Obes. Surg.*, 2005. 15(8): p. 1161-4.
[9] Cote, G.A. and S.A. Edmundowicz, Emerging technology: endoluminal treatment of obesity. *Gastrointest. Endosc.*, 2009. 70(5): p. 991-9.
[10] Mathus-Vliegen, E.M., Intragastric balloon treatment for obesity: what does it really offer? *Dig. Dis.*, 2008. 26(1): p. 40-4.
[11] Ercan, C., et al., M1363 weight reduction by means of an intragastric balloon in daily routine practice: Results at removal and in long-term. *Gastroentrol.* 2010. 138(1): p. S-389.
[12] Schwartz, M.P., et al., Endoscopic gastroplication for the treatment of gastro-oesophageal reflux disease: a randomised, sham-controlled trial. *Gut*, 2007. 56(1): p. 20-8.
[13] Fogel, R., et al., Clinical experience of transoral suturing for an endoluminal vertical gastroplasty: 1-year follow-up in 64 patients. *Gastrointest. Endosc.*, 2008. 68(1): p. 51-8.
[14] Moreno, C., et al., Transoral gastroplasty is safe, feasible, and induces significant weight loss in morbidly obese patients: results of the second human pilot study. *Endoscopy*, 2008. 40(5): p. 406-13.
[15] Familiari, P., et al., Transoral gastroplasty for morbid obesity: a multicenter trial with a 1-year outcome. *Gastrointest. Endosc.*, 2011. 74(6): p. 1248-58.
[16] Rodriguez-Grunert, L., et al., First human experience with endoscopically delivered and retrieved duodenal-jejunal bypass sleeve. *Surg. Obes. Relat. Dis.*, 2008. 4(1): p. 55-9.
[17] Cummings, D.E. and J. Overduin, Gastrointestinal regulation of food intake. *J. Clin. Invest.,* 2007. 117(1): p. 13-23.
[18] Sandler, B.J., et al., Human experience with an endoluminal, endoscopic, gastrojejunal bypass sleeve. *Surg. Endosc.*, 2011. 25(9): p. 3028-33.

Section 4: Postoperative Management

In: The Fundamentals of Bariatric Surgery
Editors: Shahzeer Karmali and Daniel W. Birch
ISBN: 978-1-62417-732-3

Chapter 13

Common Surgical Complications Following Bariatric Surgery

Esther M. Bonrath and Teodor P. Grantcharov
Division of General Surgery, St. Michael's Hospital, Toronto, ON, Canada

Abstract

A number of procedures are performed to achieve surgical weight loss. As with all interventions, each procedure carries an inherent risk of injury and thus may lead to surgical complications. The variety of different complications encountered are described in the following chapter with emphasis on morbidity and mortality rates as well as on identifying and treatment options of these surgical complications. The different risks will be discussed within the context of the individual procedures.

Introduction

A heterogeneous group of surgical procedures are performed to achieve weight-loss, these are all summarized under the category "bariatric surgery". Although pursuing the common goal of surgically altering the gastrointestinal tract in order to either reduce capacity alone or in combination with a reduction of the absorptive ability, the technical aspects do vary substantially. Due to this, besides general surgical complications, a number of specific risks for each procedure have been identified. This chapter describes common general surgical complications that may occur following bariatric surgery as well as procedure specific complication types and rates. Surgical complications can be described as being "early" (< 30 days) or "late" (> 30 days) in reference to the time of manifestation after the initial surgery. The role of surgical approach used for the procedure is frequently of relevance, therefore where applicable, data will be shown for open surgical approaches in comparison to laparoscopic approaches.

Table 1. Mortality rates for bariatric procedures

Procedure	Open surgery < 30 days	Laparoscopic surgery < 30 days
Laparoscopic adjustable gastric band (LAGB)/ Gastric banding	0.18% [4]	0 - 0.06 [1, 4, 5]
Sleeve gastrectomy (SG)	N/A	0 - 3 % [1, 6]
Gastroplasty/ vertical banded gastroplasty (VBG)	0.33% [4]	0.21% [4]
Roux-en-Y gastric bypass (RYGB)	0.4% - 0.71% [1, 4]	0.09% - 0.16% [1, 4]
Bilio-pancreatic diversion (BPD)	0.76% [4]	1.11% - 1.3% [4, 7]
Bilio-pancreatic diversion with duodenal switch (BPD-DS)	0% - 1.9% [8-10]	0% - 5% [8, 9, 11]

Table 2. Procedure specific morbidity

Procedure	Early complications (≤ 30d post-op)	Late complications (> 30d post-op)
LAGB	Gastric or esophageal perforation (0.5%) [12], port/wound infection, stoma obstruction, hemorrhage (0.1%) [12]	Band slippage (0 - 20%) [13, 14], access-port infection, port and tubing problems (2.5%) [12], band erosion (0 - 4%) [12, 14, 15]
VBG	Staple line leak, stenosis, ulcer, staple line disruption, pouch dilation and band erosion [16]	30% revision rate, anastomotic stricture, marginal ulcer, gastro-gastric fistula, bowel obstruction [16]
SG	Staple line leak (0 - 7%) [17], abscess, bleeding, stricture, splenic injury [18]	Staple line leak, stricture (0.5 - 0.9%) [6, 19]
RYGB	Anastomotic leak (0.7%) [20], gastrointestinal bleeding (0.8% - 4.4%) [21-23], bowel obstruction (0.5% - 3.3%) [16, 24]	Anastomotic stricture (3 - 27%) [25-29], bowel obstruction (1.4% - 19%) [14], marginal ulceration (4.2 - 7%) [16, 30]
BPD/ +/- DS	Abdominal hemorrhage (0.6%), leak from duodenal stump (1.5% - 7%), leak from gastric staple line (1.5%) [9], anastomotic leak (0.4%), small bowel obstruction (0.9%) [9, 31]	Incisional hernia, gastric ulcer (2 - 5%) [31], small bowel obstruction (1.3% - 2.8%) [9], malabsorption requiring lengthening of common channel (0.4%) [9]

Mortality

The overall 30-day mortality following bariatric procedures has been recorded to lie around 0.12% - 0.3% [1]. Table 1 shows the mortality rates for the most common bariatric procedures within 30 days postoperatively. Frequently, the exact cause of death remains unknown. Naturally, since this patient population may have multiple metabolic co-morbidities such as diabetes mellitus, hypertension or hypercholesterolemia they have a raised perioperative risk in comparison to healthy individuals. Data from the American Society for Metabolic and Bariatric Surgery Center of Excellence revealed that the majority of patients undergoing bariatric surgery have an ASA (American Society of Anesthesiologists) Score of ≥ 3 (RYGB 73%, LAGB 63%, SG 68%, BPD/DS 83%) [2]. Mortality may be due to major surgical complications such as anastomotic leakage or other general complications such as pulmonary embolism or cardiac events [3]. Specific surgical complications such as sepsis following enteric leaks though still remain the most frequent cause for mortality in this population [3].

General Surgical Complications

Common surgical complications can occur in all bariatric procedures; these include intra -or postoperative hemorrhage, infection, bowel obstruction or incisional hernias. The incidences of complications are associated with various procedure-specific, patient- and surgeon-related factors. The specific complications will be discussed in context of the individual procedures (Table 2).

Laparoscopic Adjustable Gastric Banding (LAGB)

The overall 30-day morbidity following LAGB (1.4%), readmission (1.7%) and reoperation rates (0.9%) are significantly lower than those of other bariatric procedures [1]. Despite this LAGB is a procedure with a number of specific mainly device-associated late complications. A late reoperation rate of 10%-20% has been described [12, 13].

Band Slippage/ Gastric Prolapse

A rate of band slippage between 0% and 20% has been described [14]. Anterior and posterior portions of the gastric fundus can be involved causing differing radiological images. This complication most frequently involves posterior slippage [32]. The associated symptoms reflect the underlying obstruction. Therefore typically regurgitation, dysphagia, reflux or pain may be described. Slippage usually occurs as a late complication. The preferred method of diagnosis is by upper gastrointestinal swallow study. This enables evaluation of the migration of the band in relation to the stomach as well as the extent of the obstruction. A severe slippage does not resolve spontaneously and should be considered an urgent event [33]. As a first measure after diagnosis deflation of the band is warranted. This may lead to rapid resolution of the symptoms and the patient can undergo elective evaluation whether revision or removal of the band is required. Seldom, the slippage can cause acute gastric wall necrosis which is generally associated with acute epigastric pain necessitating an emergent surgical approach [14, 33]. Operative possibilities to correct the slippage include salvaging the band and correcting the slippage, removing the band and placing a new one after correcting the slippage or removing the band [32, 33]. Spivak et al. 2003 [33] describe the operative approaches for a series of slippages in their patient cohort. In this study, all slippages were successfully repaired using a laparoscopic approach and all bands were salvaged. On the other hand in a series conducted in 2005 [32] of 125 slippages, 56% of patients had the band removed, 44% received repositioning or direct band replacement. Of the patients with salvaged band in this series 11% later required band removal due to recurrent slippage or erosion. The complication rate for the revision surgery was reported as 11% including complications such as gastric perforation, intraoperative hemorrhage and postoperative gastrointestinal bleeding.

Band Erosion

A rate of band erosion between 0 and 4% was reported in a systematic review conducted in 2011 [14] a further review reported an overall incidence of 1.5% with 231 erosions reported in 15,775 patients in 25 studies [15]. This typically represents a late complication. The mean time from implantation to manifestation has been reported as 12 months [15]. The most frequently described aetiology of band erosion is local ischemia due to the band's pressure on the gastric wall although a number of technical aspects appear to promote ischemia such as gastrogastric over-suturing the buckle of the band [15, 34-36]. Patients can present with unspecific abdominal pain, hematemesis, melena or simply failure to lose weight. The band eventually migrates into the stomach and then potentially can be removed endoscopically [36]. Other approaches after diagnosing band erosion without full migration including primary repair with immediate replacement [36] [12, 35], removal of band with repair [35] or conversion to an alternate bariatric procedure [37, 38].

Port Complications

A number of different complications can arise from the port and connecting tubing in LAGB. These complications are among the most common with an incidence of around 7% [39]. Access port complications frequently require operative intervention. These include flips of poorly secured ports causing inability to access the gel-chamber, this complication requires operative revision with detorquing of the flipped chamber and re-suturing the base plate securely to fascia. Another port associated problem is a leak which can occur by inadvertent puncturing the connecting tubing whilst attempting to access the port, or due to multiple punctures of the port for inflation or deflation leading to damage of the sealing gel. System leaks are common port associated complications making up to 60% of port related complications [39]. Furthermore, port infections can occur after LAGB. These can be due to a surgical site infection or contamination from port access, but late inflammatory changes over the port chamber are usually indicators of band erosion.

Roux- en Y Gastric Bypass (RYGB)

The overall rate of complications requiring reoperation following RYGB has been stated to lie around 5% with an equal incidence in open or laparoscopic approaches [1]. A number of early complications such as leaks or bleeding may require operative or interventional treatment, but also late complications such as internal hernias, stricture, gastric marginal ulcers and gastro-gastric fistulas may require further operative management and represent specific risks of RYGB.

Leaks

Gastrointestinal leaks represent the most severe complication following RYGB. A cohort evaluation of 226,456 patients revealed an incidence of enteric leak of 0.7% with an associated mortality of 6.8% [20]. Identified risk factors associated with higher risk of leak in this cohort were open gastric bypass, congestive heart failure, chronic renal failure, age older than 50 years, Medicare payer, male sex and chronic lung disease [40].

Enteric leaks can present with many different symptoms varying greatly between patients. They also represent a common cause for an extended length of hospital stay. When evaluating a postoperative patient the correct identification of an anastomotic leak may be challenging. Sustained tachycardia above 120 bpm has been shown to be a good indicator of a possible leak [41]. If other frequent causes of tachycardia such as dehydration, cardiac arrhythmias or hypoglycemia are excluded this parameter in combination with clinical judgement can be useful in deciding whether a diagnostic laparoscopy is indicated. In many cases of suspected anastomotic leak an aggressive approach with regards to second look surgery either using a laparoscopic or open approach is warranted within the early postoperative phase since other diagnostic imaging may be inconclusive and additionally defer the required operative treatment. Operative treatment should include debridement of the anastomotic leak and closure using an interrupted suture since running sutures may become loose once the inflammatory response and oedema have resolved. Revision generally includes the placement of drains at the site of the repaired leak. Depending on local findings a feeding tube may be placed in the gastric remnant to decompress the gastrointestinal tract and give an opportunity for enteric nutrition.

Bleeding

The incidence of postoperative hemorrhage has been reported as 0.8% - 4.4% [21, 23, 41]. Hemorrhage most frequently occurs from the staple lines (anastomosis or gastric pouch) but naturally can also arise from inadvert injury of spleen, liver, omentum or other abdominal structures as well as from port sites of the abdominal wall. An evaluation of acute postoperative hemorrhage showed that in most cases (60%) the bleeding was intraluminal therefore presenting with the symptoms of melena, whereas in 40% intraabdominal bleeding with the sole symptoms of tachycardia and hypovolemia was observed [23]. Of these patients only 15% required surgical treatment whilst the majority were managed conservatively [23]. A similar study by Nguyen et al 2003 [22] showed that 3.2% of patients undergoing LRYGB from their centre developed early clinical gastrointestinal hemorrhage and of these only 40% required an operative approach. Ongoing research is being conducted to optimize endoscopic staplers to reduce the risk of staple line hemorrhage. For this purpose a number of different methods such as reinforcement of the staples with biological materials [42, 43] have been pursued. Modifications of surgical technique including over-sewing or clipping staple lines are also often reported [44]. Non-operative treatment of these hemorrhages includes blood transfusion, optimizing coagulation status and endoscopy. Due to the localization of the jejunojeunostomy, endoscopically controlling bleeding from this site is far more challenging, but with sufficient expertise still can be attempted successfully.

Early Bowel Obstruction

Small bowel obstruction following bariatric surgery can occur early or late in the postoperative course. The incidence of early bowel obstruction has been shown to lie around 1.7% [45]. A variety of different aetiologies have been described. The commonest underlying mechanism is obstruction at the jejunojejunostomy. In some cases hemobezoar after intramural bleeding with hematoma have been described as causing the obstruction [45]. Early incisional hernias or internal hernias have also been associated with early small bowel obstruction, although these conditions generally manifest in the later postoperative period. Clinical presentation of early small bowel obstruction is generally with acute onset symptoms. Radiological upper gastrointestinal contrast study will be diagnostic and aid in localizing the level of obstruction. Management of this condition is ultimately determined by the underlying mechanism. Transient obstruction due to hematoma or swelling may resolve under conservative treatment, where as fixed stenosis at the jejunojejunostomy will generally require an operative approach with revision of the anastomosis. In cases of obstruction of the biliopancreatic limb massive dilatation of the gastric remenant can result which may require interventional or operative decompression. Overall though, small bowel obstruction after LRYGB represents a surgical emergency. In contrast to small bowel obstruction after other surgical procedures, even in cases with discrete symptoms, bilous vomiting and/or distended gastric remenant are symptoms that warrant an urgent operative exploration.

Stenosis/Strictures

Anastomotic strictures at the gastrojejunostomy represent common complications following RYGB. An incidence of 3% - 27% has been reported in the literature, with most of the strictures manifesting within the first few months of the procedure [25-29]. A stricture can be defined as a narrowing of the anastomosis that does not allow passage or represents significant resistance to passage of a 9-mm endoscope [46]. Factors that have been associated with an increased risk of stricture are predominantly technical aspects such as the method of anastomosis (linear, circular or hand sewn) with a higher incidence reported for circular staplers when compared to linear staplers. Additionally, the size of the stapler used has been shown to be predicative [47, 48]. For example a circular stapler size of 21 mm was shown to be an independent factor for stricture formation in a study by Takata et al. in 2007 [29].

The first treatment option for this complication especially in the early postoperative phase is an endoscopical approach. Dilatations have been shown to be the preferred method with results as high as 95% to 100% success rate with an average of 1.6 dilatations required [28, 46]. For late or refractory strictures one contributing factor that has been identified is a large-volume proximal gastric pouch [49]. Within this refractory group a surgical approach represents a good option with a reported high success rate (95%) although revisional surgery is deemed technically more challenging [49].

Marginal Ulcers

Marginal ulcers at the gastrojejunostomy are common late complications associated with RYGB. Rates vary greatly between groups (0.5% and 27%) [1, 30, 50, 51]. Multiple predisposing factors have been investigated including technical factors such method of anastomosis formation, patient related factors such as gastroesophageal reflux and peptic ulcer disease as well as helicobacter pylori infection in the patient's history. The etiology appears to be multifactorial. H. pylori infection in the history has been shown to correlate with the rate of ulceration [30], equally the type of suture used for enterotomy closure or anastomosis has been shown to influence the rate of marginal ulcers with a lower rate reported for absorbable sutures when compared to non-absorbable material (2.6% versus 1.3% [52]). The use of non-steroidal antiinflamatory drugs has also been identified as an independent risk factor [53]. The presence of gastro-gastric fistulas is also associated with a higher risk of marginal ulceration, these patients also have a higher risk of medical treatment failure requiring revisional surgery than those with ulcers alone [51, 54]. Symptoms related to marginal ulcers can remain discrete. Patients may complain of abdominal discomfort, fatigue, inability to tolerate their diet or recurrent vomiting. Some patients may present with anemia due to occult bleeding or may experience hematemsis which triggers further investigation.

Diagnosis is best made by endoscopy. Confirmation can easily be made and the extent of the ulceration validated. Figure 1 shows the endoscopic aspect of a marginal ulcer. Treatment of marginal ulcers includes medical pharmacological approaches as well as surgical options. Medical therapy with acid inhibition usually represents the initial treatment of these ulcers with good healing rates over several months of medication [30, 55]. In refractory patients or patients with diagnosed gastro-gastric fistulas revisional surgery may be required [51]. Although bariatric revisional surgery is deemed more complex and has been described as bearing more complications [56], a high success rate (87%) of a surgical approach has been described in a series of refractory patients [51].

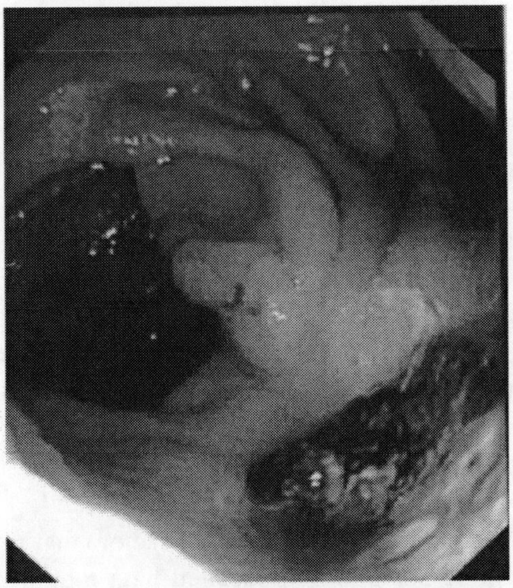

Figure 1.

Gastro-gastric Fistulas

The incidence of gastro-gastric fistulas has dramatically decreased since technical modification of the RYGB has included a complete division of the stomach rather than solely stapling without transecting. In comparison to the rate of gastro-gastric fistulas observed following VBG the numbers in RYGB are lower with recent studies reporting rates between 0.06% and 1.2% [1, 57]. The number may still be higher since this complication may remain undetected and only manifest through an inadequate weight loss. Factors that have been identified in the pathogenesis of fistula formation are incomplete transection and division of the stomach, anastomotic leaks managed conservatively, anastomotic ischemia, foreign body errosion/staples and marginal ulcers which were present in more than half of the patients evaluated in the 2005 study [57]. Gastro-gastric fistulas may lead to a vast spectrum of symptoms ranging from abdominal pain and hematomesis to more subclinical presentations with inadequate weight loss or unspecific abdominal pain [57]. Management of gastrogastric fistulas is dictated by the patient's clinical symptoms. In many cases initial treatment includes a medical approach especially when associated with a marginal ulcer. If medical treatment fails though, revisional surgery may be warranted. The need for surgery must be evaluated in context of the symptoms experienced by the patient. Possible surgical approaches include resection of the fistula and new fashioning of the gastrojejunostomy.

Late Bowel Obstructions

The incidence of late bowel obstructions in a recent review was reported as 1.4% - 19% [14]. The mean time from initial operation to presentation was 313 days in a study performed by Husain et al 2007 [58]. A number of aetiologies have been discussed that may lead to bowel obstruction following RYGB. The most frequent causes are adhesions and internal hernias. Although the rate of adhesion is related to surgical approach with a more frequent adhesion formation described following open surgery this factor could not be proven to cause obstruction in LRYGB. Literature to date rather more suggests that LRYGB either carries a higher risk of postoperative obstruction or the same risk as procedures performed in an open fashion [59-61]. These findings may be due to the higher mobility of the small bowel following laparoscopic surgery resulting in easier internal herniation.

The incidence of internal hernias has been reported as 2.1% with a mean time from procedure to necessary intervention as 413 days [62]. Common localizations of internal hernias are the transverse mesocolon, Peterson's space and the enteroenterostomy defect [62]. A number of different factors have been investigated to reduce the rate of internal hernias. So far there remains much debate about the different techniques used such as interrupted versus running suture, suture material type or even leaving all spaces open. Late internal herniation may occur despite adequate defect closure since the postoperative weight loss may lead to new defects occuring as the mesenteric fat decreases. Current randomized controlled trials on this topic are pending with results expected within the next year.

The position of the Roux limb is a well described factors that influences the rate of small bowel obstruction. A retrocolic position is associated with a higher rate of obstruction than the antecolic technique [63-65]. The position of the limb may contribute to a higher risk of herniation or compression at the level of the mesocolon. Besides internal herniation which account for approximately half of the small bowel obstructions [58], further causes include anastomotic strictures (20%), kinking of the alimentary limb (7%), incisional hernias (2%), and limb intussusception [58]. The most common symptoms associated with late small bowel obstruction following RYGB are pain (colicky in nature), nausea, vomiting, bloating and dysphagia. In a study including 2325 LRYGB procedures with a rate of small bowel obstruction of 4.4%, 82% of patients initially presented with pain as the leading symptom. Diagnostic radiology had a low sensitivity with only 48% of performed computertomographies and 55% of upper gastrointestinal series giving a positive result. In 13% of patients no radiological findings were present [58]. Since the risk of closed loop obstruction and bowel strangulation is high in these patients an early emergent operative approach, despite frequently lacking diagnostic signs on imaging is necessary even in subclinical patients. In contrast to bowel obstruction following other surgical procedures there is no role for conservative treatment in patients post LRYGB.

Sleeve Gastrectomy (SG)

The overall complication rate reported for sleeve gastrectomy lies between 0 - 29% with an average rate calculated at 9% [6]. Besides the general complications as described above a number of specific complications have been described. The reoperation and reintervention rates stated for LSG are around 3% [1].

Staple Line Leaks/Bleeding from Staple Line

A specific characteristic of the sleeve gastrectomy is the long staple line that results from transecting the stomach. Due to this, a number of concerns were initially voiced especially with regards to leak rates and bleeding from staple lines. From a review performed in 2011 the incidence of leak from a collective of 4,888 patients of was reported between 0% to 7% [17]. The hemorrhage rate was reported between 0% and 3% [17]. The majority of leaks occur at the proximal portion of the staple line with the gastroesophageal junction being identified as a special high risk zone [17]. A number of modifications in technique were trialed with the goal of reinforcing the staple line to avoid leak and bleeding, these vary greatly with regards to technique and material used. Measures such as reinforced staplers, over- sewing the staple line or buttressing with absorbable or non-absorbable material have been attempted [66-69]. A number of factors have been investigated to reduce leak risk, these include special attention to allow for tissue compression when stapling, avoidance of distal strictures to prevent a high pressure zone and avoidance of stapling too close to the gastroesophageal junction, although none of these individual factors have been proven to influence outcome in controlled trails [17]. Besides the location of the leak another important aspect is the timing of the leak especially in view of management strategies. A recent consensus paper on SG advocated the classification of leaks as acute, early, late and chronic [70]. This expert panel suggested the following terminology: acute within 7 days, early within 1-6 weeks, late after 6 weeks and chronic after 12 weeks. Current literature suggests that the majority of leaks will occur as late events leading to readmission [17, 24]. The chronic leaks may present subclinically as intraabdominal abscesses months after the initial surgery [24]. Management strategies include minimally invasive approaches with drainage as well as endoscopic management using endoluminal stents for occlusion and to dilate potential stenosis contributing to the leak. The expert consensus on this topic stated that the use of a stent represents a valid treatment option for acute proximal leaks, whereas leaks persisting after 30 days are unlikely to be successfully treated with stenting and an operative approach after 12 weeks is seen as the treatment of choice if the patient remains stable throughout this period [70]. With regards to the preferred operative approach proximal chronic leaks include revision of the sleeve and conversion to a gastric bypass [70]. Figure 2 shows the radiological findings of chronic staple line leaks with enterocutaneus fistulae following sleeve gastrectomy. Here a multimodal approach was pursued to treat this complex situation with successful intraluminal dilatation and stent treatment as well as revision surgery. Beside a more conservative approach, operative management may be required to treat persistent leaks or those leading to generalized symptoms such as abdominal sepsis and septic shock [1].

Strictures

In order to achieve satisfying results regarding weight loss SG with small residual stomachs have been preferred. This though increases the risk for the development of postoperative strictures. Currently a stricture rate of 0.5 - 0.9% has been reported [19]. Strictures following SG may be classified as early (symptomatic within the first 6 weeks following surgery) or late. The incidence of strictures can be correlated to the size of the bougie used for sleeve calibration. Current expert opinion suggests the use of a bougie between 32F and 36F. The questioned experts agreed that the use of a bougie smaller than 32 F increases the risk of complication.

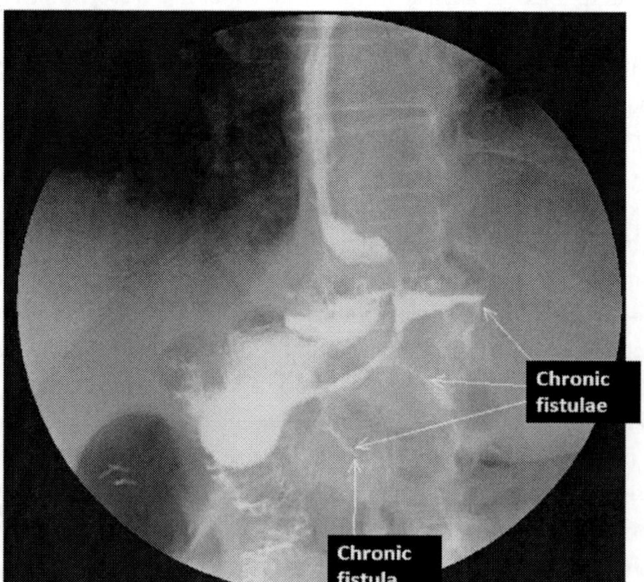

Figure 2.

Additionally the operative technique of maintaining symmetrical lateral traction whilst stapling was considered necessary in reducing stricture incidence [70]. Clinical presentation of strictures after SG is variable, and depends on the time of appearance in relation to the primary procedures and localization of the stenosis. Symptoms of acute presentation include food intolerance and vomiting once oral intake is resumed. Depending on the extent of the stenosis this may range from absolute fluid and saliva intolerance to subclinical presentations where only certain solids are not tolerated. Patients may also present with signs of increased gastroesophageal reflux or chest pain [71]. In contrast, late strictures may present with an insidious onset months after the primary procedure. In all cases, diagnostic imaging with upper gastrointestinal contrast series will demonstrate the localization and extent of the obstruction. Additionally, endoscopy is should be performed to better characterize the stricture and also offer a good interventional treatment option with a high success rate of dilatations [72]. Expert consensus with regards to treatment options included a staged approach. Four levels of implementation achieved consensus level. These include observation, endoscopic dilatation, seromyotomy and conversion to RYGB. The operative revision of the sleeve with conversion to RYGB was deemed the first treatment choice for persistent strictures that had failed an interventional apporach [70].

Biliopancreatic Diversion with or without Duodenal Switch (BPD-DS)

Biliopancreatic diversion with or without duodenal switch, combines aspects from the previously described procedures such as the sleeve gastrectomy and roux-en Y gastric bypass. A variety of different operative techniques have been trialed and are currently offered by different bariatric groups worldwide [9, 31]. The common channel in biliopancreatic diversion is far shorter than in RYGB leading to a higher level of malabsorption. The surgical complication spectrum is very similar to that encountered in the other procedures although with the incidence rates varying (Table 2). An early (< 30 days) morbidity of around 7% for major (requiring reoperation) complications has been quoted, but reports with an early morbidity as high as 28.5% have also been published [7, 9].

Operative Revision for Malnutrition

Specific aspects that need consideration are the requirement for revision surgery due to malnutrition necessitating either lengthening of the common limb or insertion of a feeding tube. In a recent series of 1000 patients who had undergone BPD-DS four patients required lengthening of the common channel in the late postoperative course (> 30 days) and a further two required the insertion of a feeding tube in order to treat malnutrition [9]. The need for an operative approach is determined by the severity of the malnutrition, intractability and associated symptoms such as diarrhoea [31]. A study conducted by Gracia et al. in 2007 showed that the need for an operative lengthening of the common channel occurred with an incidence of 2.7% in a group of patients after BPD with a common limb length of 50cm whereas none of the patients with a common limb length of 75cm required revision [7].

Furthermore severe diarrhea has been show to occur in 7 - 12% of patients depending on the exact technique employed, occasionally this can also lead to the necessity of an operative revision [31].

Leaks

With regards to postoperative leaks encountered after BPD-DS these can potential arise from the gastric staple line, duodenal stump or ileoilealanastomosis. Of the early deaths reported in series of BPD patients the most frequent cause is a enteral leakage [7, 8]. The highest incidence for leaks is found at the site of the duodenal stump (1.5 - 7%). Gastric leaks have been described as being more frequent in patients that have received an open operative approach [9]. With regards to diagnosis the same principles apply as in leaks following RYGB. In general, enteral leaks will most often require operative revision with repair and drainage which may lead to an extended length of hospital stay [7]. Additionally, intraabdominal abscesses may occur where the exact site of a leak can no longer be determined [9]. In these cases depending on the overall condition of the patient interventional drainage may be the best approach and reoperation is not always required.

Ulcers

Anastomotic ulcers may occur after BPD ±-DS. These will usually occur on the ileal side of an anastomosis, either the ileal side of a duodenoileostomy or gastroileostomy depending on the operative technique used. An incidence of 2-5% has been reported [7, 31]. Most frequently, patients present with persistent abdominal pain. An endoscopy will lead to diagnosis and should be performed. Once the diagnosis is confirmed, treatment of choice is medication with proton-pump-inhibitors. After an initial medication course of 3 months lifelong prophylaxis is suggested [31]. An operative treatment of these ulcers is not required if no complications such as bleeding or perforation occur. High recurrence rates requiring frequent endoscopic interventions and readmissions have been described in patients who did not continue PPI therapy or continued to smoke nicotine products.

Incisional Hernias

Incisional hernias can occur after any abdominal incision. In the case of BPD-DS, high rates of hernias have been described. The highest rate published stems from an open operative approach with an incidence of 50% recorded in 220 patients [7]. Similar numbers were reported by Crea et al in 2011 also for an open BPD series using two different operative modifications with a total of 504 patients [31]. This group showed an incidence of approximately 34% - 43% depending on the procedure used. In a smaller series including 43 patients comparing open versus laparoscopic BPD-DS the hernia rates were much lower with 4% in the laparotomy group and 0% in the laparoscopy group [8]. One possible explanation for the very different reported rates may be the fact that many hernias will remain asymptomatic and potentially undiscovered due to the overlying pannus. When symptomatic an operative treatment with a mesh repair is indicated after adequate weight loss, usually possible after a year following surgery. In the series reported by Jose-Antonio et al. an operative repair was usually conducted in a time frame of 18 - 24 months following surgery. This group had no hernia related complications in the interval.

Factors Influencing Morbidity and Complication Rate

A number of different factors have been investigated that have the potential to adversely influence complication rates and patient outcome. These include patient, surgeon, procedure and operative approach. These factors will be discussed within the next subsections.

Patient Factors

Data from the American Society for Metabolic and Bariatric Surgery Bariatric Surgery Center of Excellence revealed that the majority of patients undergoing bariatric surgery have a multitude of medical co-morbidities with a preoperative ASA Score of ≥ 3 [2]. This patient group is not only more challenging for the surgeon but also for the anesthetist due to a higher rate of difficult intubations. Apart from these general factors a number of patient specific risks have been identified. Patient age of 50 years or older, male gender, FEV1 <80%, have been associated with a higher risk of postoperative complications [73, 74]. On the other hand factors such as body-mass index, previous abdominal surgery and smoking still remain topic of debate [73, 74].

Surgeon Factors

The surgeon and centers expertise in the field of bariatric surgery also plays an important role in predicting patient outcome. As for a number of complex procedures, bariatric (laparoscopic) surgery has been shown to have a significant learning curve. The exact number of procedures required to achieve proficiency remains debatable. A number of studies have addressed the volume-outcome relationship on both individual and institution level. There has been a special focus on surgeon's annual volume suggesting that "high" volume surgeons have a lower morbidity and mortality rate compared with "low" volume surgeons. Despite consensus on this topic the cut-off numbers differentiating between high and low volume still remain topic of much debate [75]. Cut-off numbers such as less than 20 cases a year were correlated to an adjusted odds ratio of death of 4.7 (1.2 - 18.2) when compared to surgeons with more than 20 cases a year [76]. Another study showed similar results with an odds ratio of death of 2.5 (1.4 - 4.2) using a cut-off set at 50 cases per year [77]. The current accreditation guidelines for bariatric surgeons in fellowship according to training standards stated by the American Society for Metabolic and Bariatric Surgery (ASMBS) state that during training fellows must participate in at least 100 bariatric procedures and should have assumed the role of primary surgeon in at least 51% of cases. Following these guidelines each fellow would require a minimum of 51 bariatric cases in the fellowship year in order to be accredited by the program. Furthermore, evidence suggests that there is association between hospital volume and patient outcome indicating superior outcomes in high volume centers [75]. Research conducted to investigate the post-operative complication rate for high and low volume surgeons in high and low volume hospitals showed that high volume surgeons (>100 cases/year) operating in low volume (<150 cases/year) and high volume hospitals (>150 cases/year) had comparable complication rates which suggests that the individuals expertise plays a larger role than the expertise or volume of the centre [78].

Surgical Approach

Most bariatric groups currently aim at performing the procedures using minimally invasive approaches. Nevertheless there still remains some debate on the actual differences in morbidity with respect to the approach chosen for a procedure. Studies have demonstrated a significant higher rate of incisional hernia using an open operative approach for RYGB when compared to a laparoscopic approach (39% versus 5%) [60]. On the other hand complications such as gastrointestinal hemorrhage and small bowel obstruction have been observed more frequently in RYGB and BPD-DS in laparoscopic cohorts [9, 59]. Other complications following RYGB such as marginal ulcers have not been associated with a specific surgical approach and are equally common in open and laparoscopic groups [60]. In a recent study by Masoomi et al 2011, there was a significant higher risk of anastomotic leak in open RYGB when compared to a laparoscopic group (2.0% versus 0.3% respectively) [20]. This could also be seen in patients that received an open BPD-DS with higher leak rates at the site of the gastric staple line (1.9% versus 0%) [9]. Finally the incidence of postoperative wound infections has been shown to be associated with the approach, with a higher rate observed in patients who received an open operation [9].

Conclusion

Bariatric procedures carry an inherent risk of morbidity and mortality. These risks need to be discussed with the patient willing to undergo surgery. Morbidity has to be viewed in context of the procedure offered. Patient and surgeon factors play an important role and therefore must be addressed. Overall in comparison to other abdominal procedures, bariatric surgery is safe and effective and therefore can be offered as a good treatment option in controlling obesity and its associated co-morbidities.

References

[1] Hutter MM, Schirmer BD, Jones DB, Ko CY, Cohen ME, Merkow RP, et al. First report from the American College of Surgeons Bariatric Surgery Center Network: laparoscopic sleeve gastrectomy has morbidity and effectiveness positioned between

the band and the bypass. *Ann. Surg*. 2011;254(3):410-20; discussion 20-2. Epub 2011/08/26.

[2] DeMaria EJ, Pate V, Warthen M, Winegar DA. Baseline data from American Society for Metabolic and Bariatric Surgery-designated Bariatric Surgery Centers of Excellence using the Bariatric Outcomes Longitudinal Database. *Surgery for obesity and related diseases: official journal of the American Society for Bariatric Surgery*. 2010;6(4):347-55. Epub 2010/02/24.

[3] Smith MD, Patterson E, Wahed AS, Belle SH, Berk PD, Courcoulas AP, et al. Thirty-day mortality after bariatric surgery: independently adjudicated causes of death in the longitudinal assessment of bariatric surgery. *Obes. Surg*. 2011;21(11):1687-92. Epub 2011/08/26.

[4] Buchwald H, Estok R, Fahrbach K, Banel D, Sledge I. Trends in mortality in bariatric surgery: a systematic review and meta-analysis. *Surgery*. 2007;142(4):621-32; discussion 32-5. Epub 2007/10/24.

[5] Boza C, Gamboa C, Awruch D, Perez G, Escalona A, Ibanez L. Laparoscopic Roux-en-Y gastric bypass versus laparoscopic adjustable gastric banding: five years of follow-up. *Surgery for obesity and related diseases: official journal of the American Society for Bariatric Surgery*. 2010;6(5):470-5. Epub 2010/08/13.

[6] Gumbs AA, Gagner M, Dakin G, Pomp A. Sleeve gastrectomy for morbid obesity. *Obes. Surg*. 2007;17(7):962-9. Epub 2007/09/27.

[7] Gracia JA, Martinez M, Aguilella V, Elia M, Royo P. Postoperative morbidity of biliopancreatic diversion depending on common limb length. *Obes. Surg*. 2007;17(10): 1306-11. Epub 2007/12/22.

[8] Nelson D, Beekley A, Carter P, Kjorstad R, Sebesta J, Martin M. Early results after introduction of biliopancreatic diversion/duodenal switch at a military bariatric center. *Am. J. Surg*. 2011;201(5):678-84. Epub 2011/05/07.

[9] Biertho L, Lebel S, Marceau S, Hould FS, Lescelleur O, Moustarah F, et al. Perioperative complications in a consecutive series of 1000 duodenal switches. *Surgery for obesity and related diseases: official journal of the American Society for Bariatric Surgery*. 2011. Epub 2011/12/23.

[10] Ali MR, Fuller WD, Choi MP, Wolfe BM. Bariatric surgical outcomes. *Surg. Clin. North Am*. 2005;85(4):835-52, vii. Epub 2005/08/03.

[11] Laurenius A, Taha O, Maleckas A, Lonroth H, Olbers T. Laparoscopic biliopancreatic diversion/duodenal switch or laparoscopic Roux-en-Y gastric bypass for super-obesity-weight loss versus side effects. *Surgery for obesity and related diseases: official journal of the American Society for Bariatric Surgery*. 2010;6(4):408-14. Epub 2010/07/27.

[12] Belachew M, Belva PH, Desaive C. Long-term results of laparoscopic adjustable gastric banding for the treatment of morbid obesity. *Obes. Surg*. 2002;12(4):564-8. Epub 2002/08/27.

[13] Ponce J, Fromm R, Paynter S. Outcomes after laparoscopic adjustable gastric band repositioning for slippage or pouch dilation. *Surgery for obesity and related diseases: official journal of the American Society for Bariatric Surgery*. 2006;2(6):627-31. Epub 2006/12/02.

[14] Hamdan K, Somers S, Chand M. Management of late postoperative complications of bariatric surgery. *Br. J. Surg*. 2011;98(10):1345-55. Epub 2011/09/03.

[15] Egberts K, Brown WA, O'Brien PE. Systematic review of erosion after laparoscopic adjustable gastric banding. *Obes. Surg*. 2011;21(8):1272-9. Epub 2011/05/07.

[16] Colquitt JL, Picot J, Loveman E, Clegg AJ. Surgery for obesity. *Cochrane Database Syst. Rev*. 2009(2):CD003641. Epub 2009/04/17.

[17] Aurora AR, Khaitan L, Saber AA. Sleeve gastrectomy and the risk of leak: a systematic analysis of 4,888 patients. *Surg. Endosc*. 2011. Epub 2011/12/20.

[18] Akkary E, Duffy A, Bell R. Deciphering the sleeve: technique, indications, efficacy, and safety of sleeve gastrectomy. *Obes. Surg*. 2008;18(10):1323-9. Epub 2008/06/07.

[19] Brethauer SA, Hammel JP, Schauer PR. Systematic review of sleeve gastrectomy as staging and primary bariatric procedure. *Surgery for obesity and related diseases: official journal of the American Society for Bariatric Surgery*. 2009;5(4):469-75. Epub 2009/07/28.

[20] Masoomi H, Kim H, Reavis KM, Mills S, Stamos MJ, Nguyen NT. Analysis of factors predictive of gastrointestinal tract leak in laparoscopic and open gastric bypass. *Arch. Surg*. 2011;146(9):1048-51. Epub 2011/09/21.

[21] Higa K, Ho T, Tercero F, Yunus T, Boone KB. Laparoscopic Roux-en-Y gastric bypass: 10-year follow-up. *Surgery for obesity and related diseases: official journal of the American Society for Bariatric Surgery*. 2011;7(4):516-25. Epub 2011/02/22.

[22] Nguyen NT, Rivers R, Wolfe BM. Early gastrointestinal hemorrhage after laparoscopic gastric bypass. *Obes. Surg*. 2003;13(1):62-5. Epub 2003/03/13.

[23] Mehran A, Szomstein S, Zundel N, Rosenthal R. Management of acute bleeding after laparoscopic Roux-en-Y gastric bypass. *Obes. Surg*. 2003;13(6):842-7. Epub 2004/01/24.

[24] Kehagias I, Karamanakos SN, Argentou M, Kalfarentzos F. Randomized clinical trial of laparoscopic Roux-en-Y gastric bypass versus laparoscopic sleeve gastrectomy for the management of patients with BMI < 50 kg/m2. *Obes. Surg*. 2011;21(11):1650-6. Epub 2011/08/06.

[25] Buchwald H, Avidor Y, Braunwald E, Jensen MD, Pories W, Fahrbach K, et al. Bariatric surgery: a systematic review and meta-analysis. *JAMA*. 2004;292(14):1724-37. Epub 2004/10/14.

[26] Encinosa WE, Bernard DM, Chen CC, Steiner CA. Healthcare utilization and outcomes after bariatric surgery. *Medical care*. 2006;44(8):706-12. Epub 2006/07/25.

[27] Goitein D, Papasavas PK, Gagne D, Ahmad S, Caushaj PF. Gastrojejunal strictures following laparoscopic Roux-en-Y gastric bypass for morbid obesity. *Surg. Endosc*. 2005;19(5):628-32. Epub 2005/03/11.

[28] Nguyen NT, Stevens CM, Wolfe BM. Incidence and outcome of anastomotic stricture after laparoscopic gastric bypass. *J. Gastrointest. Surg*. 2003;7(8):997-1003; discussion Epub 2003/12/17.

[29] Takata MC, Ciovica R, Cello JP, Posselt AM, Rogers SJ, Campos GM. Predictors, treatment, and outcomes of gastrojejunostomy stricture after gastric bypass for morbid obesity. *Obes. Surg*. 2007;17(7):878-84. Epub 2007/09/27.

[30] Rasmussen JJ, Fuller W, Ali MR. Marginal ulceration after laparoscopic gastric bypass: an analysis of predisposing factors in 260 patients. *Surg. Endosc*. 2007;21(7):1090-4. Epub 2007/05/22.

[31] Crea N, Pata G, Di Betta E, Greco F, Casella C, Vilardi A, et al. Long-term results of biliopancreatic diversion with or without gastric preservation for morbid obesity. *Obes. Surg*. 2011;21(2):139-45. Epub 2010/12/01.

[32] Keidar A, Szold A, Carmon E, Blanc A, Abu-Abeid S. Band slippage after laparoscopic adjustable gastric banding: etiology and treatment. *Surg. Endosc*. 2005;19(2):262-7. Epub 2004/12/08.

[33] Spivak H, Rubin M. Laparoscopic management of lap-band slippage. *Obes. Surg*. 2003; 13(1):116-20. Epub 2003/03/13.

[34] Silecchia G, Restuccia A, Elmore U, Polito D, Perrotta N, Genco A, et al. Laparoscopic adjustable silicone gastric banding: prospective evaluation of intragastric migration of the lap-band. *Surg. Laparosc. Endosc. Percutan. Tech*. 2001;11(4):229-34. Epub 2001/08/30.

[35] Angrisani L, Di Lorenzo N, Favretti F, Furbetta F, Iuppa A, Doldi SB, et al. The Italian Group for LAP-BAND: predictive value of initial body mass index for weight loss after 5 years of follow-up. *Surg. Endosc*. 2004;18(10):1524-7. Epub 2005/03/26.

[36] Abu-Abeid S, Bar Zohar D, Sagie B, Klausner J. Treatment of intra-gastric band migration following laparoscopic banding: safety and feasibility of simultaneous laparoscopic band removal and replacement. *Obes. Surg*. 2005;15(6):849-52. Epub 2005/06/28.

[37] Himpens J, Dapri G, Cadiere GB. A prospective randomized study between laparoscopic gastric banding and laparoscopic isolated sleeve gastrectomy: results after 1 and 3 years. *Obes. Surg*. 2006;16(11):1450-6. Epub 2006/11/30.

[38] Calmes JM, Giusti V, Suter M. Reoperative laparoscopic Roux-en-Y gastric bypass: an experience with 49 cases. *Obes. Surg*. 2005;15(3):316-22. Epub 2005/04/14.

[39] Keidar A, Carmon E, Szold A, Abu-Abeid S. Port complications following laparoscopic adjustable gastric banding for morbid obesity. *Obes. Surg*. 2005;15(3):361-5. Epub 2005/04/14.

[40] Nguyen NT, Masoomi H, Laugenour K, Sanaiha Y, Reavis KM, Mills SD, et al. Predictive factors of mortality in bariatric surgery: data from the Nationwide Inpatient Sample. *Surgery*. 2011;150(2):347-51. Epub 2011/08/02.

[41] Bellorin O, Lieb J, Szomstein S, Rosenthal RJ. Laparoscopic conversion of sleeve gastrectomy to Roux-en-Y gastric bypass for acute gastric outlet obstruction after laparoscopic sleeve gastrectomy for morbid obesity. *Surgery for obesity and related diseases: official journal of the American Society for Bariatric Surgery*. 2010;6(5):566-8. Epub 2010/08/04.

[42] de la Torre RA, Scott JS. Laparoscopic Roux-en-Y gastric bypass: a totally intra-abdominal approach--technique and preliminary report. *Obes. Surg*. 1999;9(5):492-8. Epub 1999/12/22.

[43] Shikora SA, Kim JJ, Tarnoff ME. Reinforcing gastric staple-lines with bovine pericardial strips may decrease the likelihood of gastric leak after laparoscopic Roux-en-Y gastric bypass. *Obes. Surg*. 2003;13(1):37-44. Epub 2003/03/13.

[44] Higa KD, Boone KB, Ho T. Complications of the laparoscopic Roux-en-Y gastric bypass: 1,040 patients--what have we learned? *Obes. Surg*. 2000;10(6):509-13. Epub 2001/02/15.

[45] Nelson LG, Gonzalez R, Haines K, Gallagher SF, Murr MM. Spectrum and treatment of small bowel obstruction after Roux-en-Y gastric bypass. *Surgery for obesity and*

related diseases: official journal of the American Society for Bariatric Surgery. 2006;2(3):377-83, discussion 83. Epub 2006/08/24.

[46] Da Costa M, Mata A, Espinos J, Vila V, Roca JM, Turro J, et al. Endoscopic dilation of gastrojejunal anastomotic strictures after laparoscopic gastric bypass. Predictors of initial failure. *Obes. Surg.* 2011;21(1):36-41. Epub 2010/04/17.

[47] Gould JC, Garren M, Boll V, Starling J. The impact of circular stapler diameter on the incidence of gastrojejunostomy stenosis and weight loss following laparoscopic Roux-en-Y gastric bypass. *Surg. Endosc.* 2006;20(7):1017-20. Epub 2006/06/10.

[48] Nesset EM, Kendrick ML, Houghton SG, Mai JL, Thompson GB, Que FG, et al. A two-decade spectrum of revisional bariatric surgery at a tertiary referral center. *Surgery for obesity and related diseases: official journal of the American Society for Bariatric Surgery.* 2007;3(1):25-30; discussion Epub 2007/01/24.

[49] Cusati D, Sarr M, Kendrick M, Que F, Swain JM. Refractory strictures after Roux-en-Y gastric bypass: operative management. *Surgery for obesity and related diseases: official journal of the American Society for Bariatric Surgery.* 2011;7(2):165-9. Epub 2011/01/05.

[50] Huang CS, Forse RA, Jacobson BC, Farraye FA. Endoscopic findings and their clinical correlations in patients with symptoms after gastric bypass surgery. *Gastrointest Endosc.* 2003;58(6):859-66. Epub 2003/12/04.

[51] Patel RA, Brolin RE, Gandhi A. Revisional operations for marginal ulcer after Roux-en-Y gastric bypass. *Surgery for obesity and related diseases: official journal of the American Society for Bariatric Surgery.* 2009;5(3):317-22. Epub 2009/01/13.

[52] Sacks BC, Mattar SG, Qureshi FG, Eid GM, Collins JL, Barinas-Mitchell EJ, et al. Incidence of marginal ulcers and the use of absorbable anastomotic sutures in laparoscopic Roux-en-Y gastric bypass. *Surgery for obesity and related diseases: official journal of the American Society for Bariatric Surgery.* 2006;2(1):11-6. Epub 2006/08/24.

[53] Kurata JH, Nogawa AN. Meta-analysis of risk factors for peptic ulcer. Nonsteroidal antiinflammatory drugs, Helicobacter pylori, and smoking. *Journal of clinical gastroenterology.* 1997;24(1):2-17. Epub 1997/01/01.

[54] Capella JF, Capella RF. Gastro-gastric fistulas and marginal ulcers in gastric bypass procedures for weight reduction. *Obes. Surg.* 1999;9(1):22-7; discussion 8. Epub 1999/03/05.

[55] Hedberg J, Hedenstrom H, Nilsson S, Sundbom M, Gustavsson S. Role of gastric acid in stomal ulcer after gastric bypass. *Obes. Surg.* 2005;15(10):1375-8. Epub 2005/12/16.

[56] Brolin RE, Cody RP. Impact of technological advances on complications of revisional bariatric operations. *J. Am. Coll. Surg.* 2008;206(3):1137-44. Epub 2008/05/27.

[57] Carrodeguas L, Szomstein S, Soto F, Whipple O, Simpfendorfer C, Gonzalvo JP, et al. Management of gastrogastric fistulas after divided Roux-en-Y gastric bypass surgery for morbid obesity: analysis of 1,292 consecutive patients and review of literature. *Surgery for obesity and related diseases: official journal of the American Society for Bariatric Surgery.* 2005;1(5):467-74. Epub 2006/08/24.

[58] Husain S, Ahmed AR, Johnson J, Boss T, O'Malley W. Small-bowel obstruction after laparoscopic Roux-en-Y gastric bypass: etiology, diagnosis, and management. *Arch. Surg.* 2007;142(10):988-93. Epub 2007/10/17.

[59] Podnos YD, Jimenez JC, Wilson SE, Stevens CM, Nguyen NT. Complications after laparoscopic gastric bypass: a review of 3464 cases. *Arch. Surg*. 2003;138(9):957-61. Epub 2003/09/10.

[60] Puzziferri N, Austrheim-Smith IT, Wolfe BM, Wilson SE, Nguyen NT. Three-year follow-up of a prospective randomized trial comparing laparoscopic versus open gastric bypass. *Ann. Surg*. 2006;243(2):181-8. Epub 2006/01/25.

[61] Smith SC, Edwards CB, Goodman GN, Halversen RC, Simper SC. Open vs laparoscopic Roux-en-Y gastric bypass: comparison of operative morbidity and mortality. *Obes. Surg*. 2004;14(1):73-6. Epub 2004/02/26.

[62] Ahmed AR, Rickards G, Husain S, Johnson J, Boss T, O'Malley W. Trends in internal hernia incidence after laparoscopic Roux-en-Y gastric bypass. *Obes. Surg*. 2007;17(12): 1563-6. Epub 2007/11/16.

[63] Hwang RF, Swartz DE, Felix EL. Causes of small bowel obstruction after laparoscopic gastric bypass. *Surg. Endosc*. 2004;18(11):1631-5. Epub 2005/06/03.

[64] Cho M, Carrodeguas L, Pinto D, Lascano C, Soto F, Whipple O, et al. Diagnosis and management of partial small bowel obstruction after laparoscopic antecolic antegastric Roux-en-Y gastric bypass for morbid obesity. *J. Am. Coll. Surg*. 2006;202(2):262-8. Epub 2006/01/24.

[65] Felsher J, Brodsky J, Brody F. Small bowel obstruction after laparoscopic Roux-en-Y gastric bypass. *Surgery*. 2003;134(3):501-5. Epub 2003/10/14.

[66] Cottam D, Qureshi FG, Mattar SG, Sharma S, Holover S, Bonanomi G, et al. Laparoscopic sleeve gastrectomy as an initial weight-loss procedure for high-risk patients with morbid obesity. *Surg. Endosc*. 2006;20(6):859-63. Epub 2006/06/02.

[67] Roa PE, Kaidar-Person O, Pinto D, Cho M, Szomstein S, Rosenthal RJ. Laparoscopic sleeve gastrectomy as treatment for morbid obesity: technique and short-term outcome. *Obes. Surg*. 2006;16(10):1323-6. Epub 2006/10/25.

[68] Dapri G, Cadiere GB, Himpens J. Reinforcing the staple line during laparoscopic sleeve gastrectomy: prospective randomized clinical study comparing three different techniques. *Obes. Surg*. 2010;20(4):462-7. Epub 2009/12/17.

[69] Consten EC, Gagner M. Staple-line reinforcement techniques with different buttressing materials used for laparoscopic gastrointestinal surgery: a new strategy to diminish perioperative complications. *Surgical technology international*. 2004;13:59-63. Epub 2005/03/04.

[70] Rosenthal RJ, Diaz AA, Arvidsson D, Baker RS, Basso N, Bellanger D, et al. International Sleeve Gastrectomy Expert Panel Consensus Statement: best practice guidelines based on experience of >12,000 cases. *Surgery for obesity and related diseases: official journal of the American Society for Bariatric Surgery*. 2012;8(1):8-19. Epub 2012/01/18.

[71] Zundel N, Hernandez JD, Galvao Neto M, Campos J. Strictures after laparoscopic sleeve gastrectomy. *Surg. Laparosc. Endosc. Percutan. Tech*. 2010;20(3):154-8. Epub 2010/06/17.

[72] Lalor PF, Tucker ON, Szomstein S, Rosenthal RJ. Complications after laparoscopic sleeve gastrectomy. *Surgery for obesity and related diseases: official journal of the American Society for Bariatric Surgery*. 2008;4(1):33-8. Epub 2007/11/06.

[73] Gonzalez R, Bowers SP, Venkatesh KR, Lin E, Smith CD. Preoperative factors predictive of complicated postoperative management after Roux-en-Y gastric bypass for morbid obesity. *Surg. Endosc.* 2003;17(12):1900-4. Epub 2003/10/10.
[74] Nguyen NT, Rivers R, Wolfe BM. Factors associated with operative outcomes in laparoscopic gastric bypass. *J. Am. Coll. Surg.* 2003;197(4):548-55; discussion 55-7. Epub 2003/10/03.
[75] Zevin B, Aggarwal R, Grantcharov T. Volume-outcome association in bariatric surgery: A systematic review. *Ann Surg*. 2012. Epub Ahead of print.
[76] Flum DR, Dellinger EP. Impact of gastric bypass operation on survival: a population-based analysis. *J. Am. Coll. Surg.* 2004;199(4):543-51. Epub 2004/09/30.
[77] Campos GM, Ciovica R, Rogers SJ, Posselt AM, Vittinghoff E, Takata M, et al. Spectrum and risk factors of complications after gastric bypass. *Arch. Surg.* 2007;142(10):969-75; discussion 76. Epub 2007/10/17.
[78] Weller WE, Rosati C, Hannan EL. Relationship between surgeon and hospital volume and readmission after bariatric operation. *J. Am. Coll. Surg.* 2007;204(3):383-91. Epub 2007/02/28.

In: The Fundamentals of Bariatric Surgery
Editors: Shahzeer Karmali and Daniel W. Birch
ISBN: 978-1-62417-732-3

Chapter 14

Nutritional Follow-up of the Bariatric Patient Postoperative

Carlene Johnson Stoklossa and Janet Stadnyk
Nutrition Services, Alberta Health Services, Edmonton, Alberta, Canada

Abstract

Treatment for morbid obesity, including bariatric surgery, is more successful when multidisciplinary health care providers assess, treat, monitor and evaluate individuals both before and after surgery. To achieve and maintain health benefits and weight loss after bariatric surgery, significant and lifelong lifestyle changes are required. Important outcomes of bariatric surgery include improvement or resolution of co-morbid conditions and improved quality of life.

Bariatric surgery has a significant impact on nutritional status. Nutrition care by a registered dietitian is recommended before and after bariatric surgery as part of a comprehensive weight management treatment plan. This chapter provides an overview of the nutrition care for patients after bariatric surgery based upon available evidence and best/promising practice. Surgical procedures and their nutritional impact are outlined. Nutrition care, including intervention, monitoring and evaluation are reviewed. A post operative fluid diet is started immediately following surgery and is later progressed to a solid diet with modifications to accommodate the gut alterations and individual tolerance. Recommendations for a long term diet including life-long vitamin and mineral supplementation are described. Nutrition monitoring and evaluation after bariatric surgery include weight, diet, and blood work, eating behaviours and vitamin and mineral supplementation. Nutritional management of potential complications, including dumping syndrome are reviewed.

Introduction

Obesity is a complex chronic disease with many contributory factors. Treatment with lifestyle and medication interventions can produce modest but clinically significant improvements in health and weight status. Outcomes may not be sufficient to reduce health risk and long-term success is limited. Bariatric surgery is the most efficacious treatment available for obesity, improving co-morbid conditions, achieving greater weight loss and improved sustainability in most individuals. [1, 2, 3]

Bariatric surgery refers to a number of different surgical interventions that support weight management and related co-morbid conditions for those with morbid obesity. There are three main types of bariatric surgical procedures which can be defined by function: restrictive, combined (restrictive and malabsorptive) and primarily malabsorptive [4]. Each procedure assists with weight management by restricting food intake. Some procedures may also produce malabsorption by altering the gastrointestinal tract. All procedures have an impact on nutritional status [5]. The following is a brief overview of the surgeries and their nutritional impact.

Bariatric Surgical Procedures and Nutritional Impact

Restrictive Procedures

Vertical Banded Gastroplasty (VBG) [6] and *Laparoscopic Adjustable Gastric Band (LAGB)* [6] procedures create a small pouch (approximately 30 mL volume or the size of a thumb) and a narrowed opening or stoma (up to 10 mm or the size of a dime) into the main stomach. The remainder of the stomach is intact with no alterations to the intestine, leaving digestion and absorption unchanged. The first effect is to produce fullness and satiety with a smaller portion of solid food (e.g. approximately 1 cup [250 mL]). The second effect is to delay emptying of food from the pouch into the stomach through the narrow opening/stoma with a fixed (VBG) or adjustable (LAGB) band, prolonging satiety. The LAGB reservoir is inflated with a saline solution through a port secured to the abdominal wall. The adjustment is customized to each individual to create appropriate narrowing of the stoma to produce sufficient early satiety and assist with sustaining weight reduction.

Sleeve Gastrectomy (SG): [2, 7, 8, 9, 10, 11, 12] Rather than a pouch, this procedure creates a "sleeve" in the stomach, extending from the esophagus to the duodenum. The size of the gastric sleeve is approximately 60 to 120 mL. The gastric remnant, approximately 80 % of the stomach, is removed. Production of grehlin, a hormone involved in appetite, is reduced, resulting in decreased hunger and improved satiety. No alterations are made to the intestine, leaving absorption of food unchanged. However, reduction of stomach acid and removal of parietal cell mass may impact digestion and absorption of iron, calcium and vitamin B_{12}.

Combined Procedures

Roux-En-Y Gastric Bypass (RYGB) procedure creates a small gastric pouch (30 mL) by stapling and dividing the stomach. Next, the small intestine is dissected at about 100 to 150 cm from the stomach. The distal end is attached to the pouch and the proximal end is re-attached to the small intestine. All oral intake completely bypasses the stomach and duodenum, emptying directly into the jejunum. Digestion and absorption of iron, calcium, folic acid and vitamin B_{12} are impacted. Dumping syndrome can occur with this procedure.

The Biliopancreatic Diversion with or without Duodenal Switch (BPD +/- DS) procedure combines removal of a small section of stomach with the alterations to the path of the small intestine. Complication rates are higher and include malabsorption, foul smelling stools, flatus, protein malnutrition, vitamin and mineral deficiencies, anemia, osteoporosis and anastomotic ulceration. [1] Dumping syndrome can occur with this procedure.

Malabsorptive Procedures

Malabsorptive procedures decrease absorption of nutrients by decreasing the length of small intestine that is exposed to food. The *Jejunoileal Bypass (JIB)* is a procedure that bypasses most of the small intestine, leaving a very short length (about 35 cm) of small bowel for absorption. Malabsorptive procedures produce significant weight loss but also have the highest complication rates, such as organ (liver, kidney) failure and mortality. Malabsorption of both macronutrients and micronutrients contribute to severe malnutrition and related complications. All individuals should be considered at high risk for malnutrition. This procedure is no longer recommended due to significantly high complication rates. [2, 1, 13]

Nutrition Care after Bariatric Surgery

A description of key components of nutrition assessment is provided in Chapter 3. Nutrition care after bariatric surgery is a continuation of the pre-surgical care. This section will review the nutrition follow up including recommendations for post-surgery diets, vitamins and minerals and blood work.

Routine postoperative follow up appointments with the registered dietitian are scheduled at points where specific nutrition intervention, monitoring or evaluation is required, but may be altered based on individual patient progress or complications. The following post-operative routine is recommended for routine nutrition intervention, monitoring and evaluation: prior to discharge from the hospital, 1-2 weeks, 1, 2, 3, 6, 9 months then annually. [5, 14] Anthropometric measurements are taken at each visit, including weight and BMI. Assessment of the total weight loss and rate of weight change is important to evaluate and adjust interventions. Routine blood work including vitamin levels is recommended within 6 months and annually post surgery. Pre-surgical blood work provides a reference point for comparison to post-surgical values. More frequent monitoring may be required for deficiencies, patients who are not taking supplements as recommended or with changes to health status. [5]

Patients should be encouraged to continue with a self- monitoring journal for their own benefit and assist with communication of progress at each follow-up visit. Patients experience many changes following bariatric surgery and keeping a journal helps patients effectively self-manage their health. The information gathered is invaluable to post operative care, providing information related to intake, activity, symptoms, weight status, emotions or stress levels. The journal can help patients self manage their symptoms and work together with their health care provider to achieve their goals.

The registered dietitian should assess intake of fluid, protein, calories, appropriateness of food choices, portions and eating patterns. After bariatric surgery, all patients should be monitored for protein-energy malnutrition which can occur and is primarily the result of inadequate intake. [15] Barriers to adequate oral intake may include changes in taste preferences, hunger, thirst, difficulty swallowing larger volumes of fluids and lactose intolerance. A review of food intake should evaluate if there is selection of inappropriate foods, food consistencies or portion sizes. This information is especially important to inform treatment decisions related to adjustments to the laparoscopic adjustable gastric bands. Proactively monitoring and supporting the patient to follow post operative diet guidelines is important to ensure optimal efficacy of the gastric band.

Post Operative Diet

Evidence-based standardized protocols for diet after bariatric surgeries are not available. The following is a review of diet recommendations based upon available evidence and best practice

Fluid Diet

A liquid diet is provided in the immediate post operative period. The rationale for providing a liquid diet after surgery is to decrease irritation of the surgical site while it is healing and reduce risk of emesis. It is important ensure the diet provide adequate fluid to prevent dehydration. The total volume of fluids consumed at one time is small as to avoid overfilling or blockage of the new stomach pouch, causing discomfort, vomiting and heartburn. The fluid diet also needs to provide adequate protein for wound healing, to promote satiety and to limit loss of muscle during weight loss. Total caloric intake should be sufficient to meet carbohydrate and protein requirements and limited to promote weight loss.

Practices vary with many centres using a clear fluid diet prior to initiation of a full fluid diet in the immediate post-operative period. There is some evidence that a clear fluid diet may not be required. [16] A clear fluid diet is nutritionally inadequate so if initiated, should not be continued for more than 24-48 hours. Some centres use a staged diet approach, where Stage 1 is a clear fluid diet. [5]

The Full Fluid Bariatric Diet (Stage II) is recommended for approximately 14 days after surgery while the stomach is healing and swelling is decreasing. Length of time may vary, depending on the assessment of the surgeon and registered dietitian to determine when it is appropriate for the patient to advance with solid foods. Food and beverages that are permitted on the Full Fluid Bariatric diet are summarized in Table 1. Rationale for items included is that they should be liquid or melt at room temperature, can be poured, have a pureed or baby food texture and do not contain any solid pieces of food.

Carbonated beverages are generally not recommended anytime after bariatric surgery. The gas may contribute to distention of the pouch, leading to discomfort, heartburn, vomiting and possible increase of compliancy (i.e. the distention of a hollow organ to accommodate a volume [17]) of the gastric pouch. There is a lack evidence to support or dispute recommendations for carbonation after bariatric surgery.

Caffeine is not recommended during the first few weeks to reduce possible gastric irritation to the new surgical site. Caffeine is allowed on the post surgical diet (within recommended amounts) when healing has occurred and the diet is advanced to solid foods.

Calories

Adequate calories are required to meet minimum carbohydrate (DRI 130 grams per day) and protein requirements (see next section). Daily intake should target a 500-1000 kcal reduction from total daily energy requirements to promote weight loss. However, due to the functional restriction after bariatric surgery, total volume of intake is limited. In the first few weeks after surgery, the total caloric intake is usually very low (e.g. 800-1200 kcal per day).

Carbohydrate and calorie intake is limited primarily by portion size due to volume limitations of the small gastric pouch or sleeve. The exclusive use of sugar-free or calorie-reduced products is not suitable for this intervention as these products may further reduce the total caloric intake below recommendations (e.g. 300-500 kcal/day). Inadequate caloric intake and hypoglycemia may result.

Protein

An estimated protein requirement to promote wound healing and minimize loss of lean muscle mass during weight loss is 1-1.2 grams/kg ideal body weight (ideal = BMI 24.9 kg/m^2). Most individuals will not be able to meet their protein needs with the foods permitted on Full Fluids Bariatric diet alone so a protein supplement is required. Supplements that provide a good source of protein (whey or soy) without excess calories or vitamins are recommended. Protein-only supplements (e.g. skim milk powder, commercial protein powders or liquid protein) can be mixed into food or drinks to increase the protein content. Meal replacement products can provide a good source of protein and vitamins, but also contain extra calories. If meal replacement products are recommended, a nutrition prescription indicating the specific amount of each product to meet protein needs and prevent excess caloric intake should be provided. Protein bars and other solid foods should be avoided at this time.

Fluid

Fluid intake should meet daily requirements, be sufficient to satisfy thirst and produce adequate urine output. A practical method to achieve this is to recommend 125 mL fluid intake every hour while awake. Fluids should be sipped slowly from a cup or a glass. Consuming fluids from a straw or sports-bottle can increase the rate and amount of intake or contribute to swallowing of air resulting in discomfort, vomiting or heartburn. In general, it is important to educate the individual to take small sips of fluid and stop when they start to feel full, heaviness or pressure.

Table 1. Full Fluid Bariatric Diet

Food Group	Choose	Avoid
Grain Products	Thin hot cereal, oatmeal, oat bran, Cream of Wheat®, cream of rice or infant cereals	All other Grain products
Vegetables and Fruit	juice, 100% pure vegetable or fruit- limit to ½ cup per day	All other Vegetables and Fruits
	applesauce or other pureed fruit, unsweetened	
Milk and Alternatives	milk, skim or 1% or lactose-reduced milk, fortified soy or rice beverage	Cheese, cottage cheese
	yogurt, low fat or fat free (no fruit pieces)	Any product with any added food listed as Avoid (fruit, cereal, nuts, seeds)
	yogurt drinks, low fat or fat free(no fruit pieces)	
	pudding or custard, made with low fat milk	
Meat and Alternatives	tofu (soy), soft or silken	All other Meat and Alternatives
Fats and Oils	liquid vegetable oils, margarine	Nuts, seeds, peanut and other nut butters
Drinks	Coffee or tea, herbal or caffeine-free	Caffeine
	Water	Alcohol
	Low calorie beverages like Crystal Lite®, fruit-flavoured waters, diet iced tea, diet lemonade	Drinks with added sugar Carbonated Drinks
Other Foods	Soup, strained, blended or broth	Soup with noodles, rice, vegetables or meat
	Jell-0®	Jell-O® with added Fruit
	Popsicles or low calorie frozen dessert made with artificial sweetener	Frozen desserts with added sugar, high fat, fruit or nuts
Supplements	Protein supplements (liquid or powder)	Protein bars

Progression to Solid Foods

There are no evidenced-based standardized protocols for the progression from a liquid diet to the introduction of solid foods after bariatric surgery. Individuals are advised to follow a well-balanced, calorie-reduced diet as part of a comprehensive weight management strategy. Practice is variable and may include several different diet stages and texture progressions. On average, advancement texture from fluids to solid foods, or Stage III, occurs about 2 to 4 weeks after surgery. [5, 6] Best practice recommendations include consuming small portions, consuming liquids separate from solids, avoiding certain textures and an emphasis on meeting protein requirements. Assessment is required by the surgeon and registered dietitian to determine when it is appropriate to advance to solid foods for an individual.

Calories

Individual assessment is required to determine appropriate caloric requirements based on the individual's health and weight status. Daily intake should provide adequate calories to meet minimum carbohydrate (130 grams/day [18]) and protein requirements (see next section) and up to 500-1000 kcal reduction from total daily energy requirements to promote weight loss and enhance prevention of weight gain.

Protein

The goal is to provide adequate protein for wound healing, promote satiety and limit loss of muscle during weight loss. An estimated protein requirement to minimize loss of lean muscle mass during weight loss is 1-1.2 g/kg IBW. Intakes of 1.5g/kg IBW may exceed requirements for non-complicated individuals and displace other nutrients with volume restrictions and lower calorie intakes after surgery. [5] A protein supplement may be required to meet requirements when advancing from fluids to solid foods. Supplements that provide a good source of protein (whey or soy) without excess calories or vitamins are recommended if required to meet both calorie and protein goals. As there are many products available, all supplements should be reviewed and recommended by the registered dietitian. Once tolerating solid foods, protein requirement can often be met without the use of supplements.

Fluid

Fluid intake should meet daily requirements, be sufficient to satisfy thirst and produce adequate urine output. Fluid requirements do not change after bariatric surgery, but achieving these targets can be challenging. Individuals need to separate liquid intake from solid food to avoid overfilling of the pouch leading to vomiting or rapid emptying of the pouch leading to lack of satiety and increased intake. Individuals need education and regular support to take small sips of fluids throughout the day. If they wait until they are thirsty, then try to drink a larger amount of fluid, they will often experience discomfort and emesis. Fluids should be sipped slowly from a cup or a glass. Consuming fluids from a straw or sports-bottle type lid can increase the rate and amount of intake or contribute to swallowing of air resulting in discomfort, vomiting and/or heartburn. As previously mentioned carbonated beverages should be avoided as they are thought to be a contributing factor to increased compliance of the gastric pouch over time and may cause vomiting and discomfort.

Fluids should not be consumed within 30 minutes (before or after) of eating any solid foods. Beverages and liquid foods (e.g. soup) should be consumed between meals and snacks. Limit the amount of fluids consumed at one time to avoid overfilling or blockage of the new stomach pouch, causing discomfort, vomiting and heartburn.

Meal Frequency

The recommended meal frequency is the same for non-surgical weight management. Meals should occur three times per day, including breakfast plus 1 to 2 small snacks. Some individuals may need to eat more often (e.g. have 3 snacks) to meet nutritional requirements, especially if total volume of solid food tolerated is small.

Portion Control and Satiety

Individuals should start with small portions of solid foods (e.g. approximately ¼ cup [60 mL] or "two bites"), advancing to small meals and snacks (e.g. limit solid food to approximately 1 cup [250 mL] at each meal or snack). The total volume of food tolerated varies between patients and can also depend on the food selected, eating environment or time of day.

Food texture has an impact on satiety. Solid foods will contribute to early satiety and reduction of total volume ingested which promotes weight loss. Liquids and semi-solid foods will empty from the pouch or sleeve faster than solids, so are less satiating than solids. As a result, individuals consuming liquids or semi-solids may experience an early return of hunger and as a result increased intake.

It is important to eat slowly, chew foods well and build awareness for the early signs of fullness to prevent discomfort and vomiting. Patients should be educated to make time for meals and snacks to eat slowly (e.g.15 to 30 minutes) and to be mindful when eating (e.g. not eating while distracted by watching TV, driving or working). It is important to educate the individual to stop eating or drinking when they *start* to feel a fullness, heaviness or pressure in the pouch/sleeve. They should not continue to eat or try to finish their serving as they may overfill the pouch leading to discomfort, heartburn, burping or vomiting. Patients should be educated to use internal cues for satiety and fullness, rather than external cues such as the portion on their plate.

Over time, individuals may report a decreased sensation of fullness with the portion of solid food that previously provided satiety. They may increase their portions to achieve the sensation of fullness, leading to increased total caloric intake and possibly further increase in compliancy of the pouch. Counseling provided to patients pre-operatively to manage portion sizes can be reinforced postoperatively for lifelong weight management.

Food Choices, Texture and Tolerance

Multiple factors impact both the quantity and quality of intake after bariatric surgery. Recommendations should be consistent with general healthy eating guidelines, cardio-protective nutrition guidelines, bariatric surgery and weight management principles. For individual education, a detailed list of foods described as " Not Recommended" may be provided. It is important to avoid the terms "good" and "bad" when discussing food choices to promote a balanced approach to healthy eating and avoid the "all or nothing" approach with individuals. Portion sizes are variable based on individual tolerance, preferences and nutrition recommendations.

Table 2. Food and Drink Choices Not Recommended due to Texture

Not Recommended	Explanation
Vegetables and Fruit	
Fried vegetables (e.g. zucchini, French fries)	Crisp outside, soft inside texture may be difficult to chew well
Fruit; dried or leathers	Sticky texture, difficult to chew well
Skin, peel or seeds of some vegetables and fruits	Difficult to chew well
Grains	
Rice and dishes made with rice	Difficult to chew well, Sticky texture; may stick together in pouch
Pyroghy, dumpling or steam buns	Sticky texture, may stick together in pouch
Breads; soft, fluffy type	Soft texture, sticky. Better tolerated if toasted
Grain Products containing nuts or dried fruits (e.g. raisin bread) including granola or trail mix	May swallow dried fruit or nut without chewing well, causing discomfort and possible blockage of stoma or outlet of gastric band
Cereal or energy bars, chewy-style	Sticky texture
Popcorn	Difficult to chew well for some people
Muffins	Soft, doughy texture, may stick together in pouch
Meat and Alternatives	
Battered or deep fried choices	Difficult to chew well with crisp outside, soft inside
Chicken wings	Difficult to chew well, especially with skin
Meat (e.g. steak, roast or chop)	Difficult to chew well due to muscle fibres, even if tender. Ground meat may be better tolerated.
Meats with a casing: sausage, smokies, wieners/hot dogs, pepperoni sticks	Difficult to chew well
Tough or dry cuts of meat and jerky	Difficult to chew well.
Skin of poultry or fish	Difficult to chew well
Milk and Milk Products	
Rice pudding	Sticky texture
Supplements	
Some protein or energy bars	Sticky dense texture, difficult to chew well
Beverages	
Carbonated drinks (regular or diet products)	Trigger for nausea, burping or emesis May lead to increased pouch compliancy
Other: Gummy candy	Sticky texture, difficult to chew well

After bariatric surgery, the term "tolerance" is used to describe foods that the person has the ability to chew well into very small pieces, permitting a comfortable feeling of fullness and the food to pass through the stoma without discomfort. If a food is "poorly tolerated", it does not pass through the opening of the stoma. This is often because it is difficult to chew well or has a soft or sticky texture. If foods are poorly tolerated, signs and symptoms may include heartburn, burping, discomfort (described as heaviness or pressure), feelings of food being "stuck" and vomiting. Key behaviours that lead to poor tolerance are eating too fast, eating too much, food not chewed adequately, consumption of a food not recommended or eating while distracted. Refer to Table 3 for other nutrition-related behaviours that may cause problems after bariatric surgery.

Not Recommended foods (see Table 2) are classified as such listed due to physical properties (e.g. textural issues or carbonation) or nutrient quality (e.g. high sugar, fat, sodium). The texture of certain items may be difficult to chew well (e.g. red meat) leading to nausea, heartburn, discomfort and vomiting. Patients should be educated to avoid certain food and drinks that are poorly tolerated, increasing risk of emesis and possible obstruction or irritation of the stoma.

If an individual is able to tolerate certain foods listed as "Not Recommended" and considered a healthy option (e.g. rice, skin or peel of vegetables) it is acceptable to include as part of their intake. Individuals may be able to tolerate certain foods that are not considered a healthy option (e.g. potato chips), however these foods remain "Not Recommended" due to high in fat, sugar, sodium or caloric content.

Table 3. Common Nutrition-Related Behaviours after Bariatric Surgery

Taste changes • Increased sensitivity or acuity to sweet • Aversion to meat
Difficulty tolerating or advancing to solid foods • Fear of initiation of food or drink right after surgery • Fear of advancement to solid foods. • Prefers ease of drinking fluids versus preparing or chewing solid food. • Experiences intolerance of a food early after surgery, now avoids this food long term. Early intolerances may not persist.
Choosing foods that are easy to chew and easily digestible • Foods with a crisp texture that can break down easily (e.g. potato chips). Even if these food choices are small in portion, they are calorically dense and nutrient-poor.
Lack of variety • Fear of intolerance leading to individuals selecting a narrow range of items (only "safe" foods) that are well tolerated.
Grazing behaviour • Consumption of small portions prevents overfilling of pouch, discomfort and a lack of connection to fullness-hunger signal • Unable to complete portion at meal, so they "pick at it" over the next hour or two. May contribute to excess total calories • Lack of time management to take time for meals and breaks to eat slowly, chew well.
Choosing liquids with solids • Taking sips of fluids to help food pass through the pouch, increasing portions (Reported as a technique used when eating in public place (e.g. work, social event) to help prevent blockage, emesis or help avoid comments as to why the person is eating such a small portion.) • Using excess condiments to help lubricate food, permitting easy passage through the pouch. • Choosing foods with a fluid or semi solid textures more often, limited intake of solid food. This may contribute to excess total calories

Many of these items are easy to chew and digest and are calorically dense, which may contribute to excess caloric intake. These foods are not consistent with cardio-protective nutrition guidelines and may also contribute to complications (e.g. dumping syndrome after gastric bypass).

Vitamins and Minerals

Bariatric surgery increases the risk for vitamin and mineral deficiencies. [5, 24, 19] This may be due to:

- decreased intake due to smaller stomach size
- decreased intake due to intolerance of certain foods or textures
- malabsorption (for some procedures)
- lack of knowledge or education regarding nutritional impact of bariatric surgery and recommendations
- lack of adherence to nutrition recommendations
- co-morbid conditions
- drug-nutrient interactions

After bariatric surgery, all individuals require multivitamin and mineral supplementation and monitoring. The type and dose will vary depending on the type of surgery in addition to the age, gender and health of the individual. Vitamin and mineral supplements are required for life as individuals cannot meet their requirements from diet alone.

Restrictive Procedures (LAGB/VBG)

The risk for vitamin and mineral deficiencies is lower for this type of surgery as digestion and absorption is not impaired. However, avoidance of certain foods and limited intake of food due to small portions can increase the risk of deficiencies. Supplementation recommendations include one multivitamin and mineral supplement daily and meeting calcium and vitamin D requirements for age, gender and health conditions.

Table 4. Alternative Formats for Vitamin and Mineral Supplements

Tablet form	Alternative Suggestion
Multivitamin and Mineral	Adult chewable (children's formulations are often inadequate in composition)
Prenatal multivitamin	PregVit® (2 small pills) or adult chewable plus the addition of other vitamins/minerals to meet amounts provided by the prenatal (e.g. iron/folate)
Calcium	Liquid, chewable tablet (avoid soft chews due to sticky texture, may block stoma)
Vitamin D	Liquid, drops, Injection(see physician)
Vitamin B_{12}	Fast dissolve strip(on the tongue), sublingual tablet, Injection(see physician)
Iron	Liquid, Injection-(see physician)

Sleeve Gastrectomy (SG)

There is very limited research on the short term nutritional implications of this surgery and no long term data. There is an increased risk of iron, calcium and vitamin B_{12} deficiencies with this surgery due to the resection of the majority of the stomach, reducing stomach acid and intrinsic factor. Current best practice recommends the same vitamin and mineral supplementation as gastric bypass with monitoring and evaluation of micronutrient status. Further research is required.

Malabsorptive Procedures (JIB, BPD)

Malabsorptive procedures decrease absorption of nutrients by decreasing the length of small intestine that is exposed to food, resulting in malnutrition and several vitamin and mineral deficiencies. There is a higher risk of vitamin and mineral deficiencies uncommon in other bariatric procedures including vitamins A, E, K, selenium and zinc. Monitoring and evaluation of serum values can provide guidance for supplementation for all vitamins and minerals.

Roux-En-Y Gastric Bypass (RYGB)

Incidences of malnutrition and vitamin/mineral deficiencies are higher due to the malabsorptive component for gastric bypass. Nutrients of concern include calcium and vitamin D, vitamin B_{12}, folic acid, iron and thiamine. A pregnancy multivitamin provides higher amounts of iron, calcium, vitamin B_{12} and folic acid than a standard adult multivitamin. One prenatal multivitamin daily is recommended for both men and women.

A daily target of 1500-2000 mg elemental calcium is prescribed; taking in consideration that calcium absorption is compromised. Combined diet and supplement intake of calcium >1700 mg/day is thought to prevent bone loss during weight loss. [25] Calcium citrate is the preferred calcium supplement to optimize absorption in a low acid environment. Calcium supplement recommendations are generally1200 to1500 mg of elemental calcium daily so that in combination with the oral diet, the daily target of 1500-2000 mg elemental calcium is met.

It is recommended to take a combined supplement of calcium with vitamin D to assist absorption and reduce the number of tablets required each day. Vitamin D supplement recommendations should be targeted to keep serum levels within normal limits for the individual (see Chapter 3).

Multivitamin and Mineral Supplements

Multivitamin and mineral supplements should be complete and include selenium and zinc. [24] Deficiencies in zinc, selenium, vitamin A, E and C are rare but have been reported. They are more common with malabsorptive procedures, but may occur with lack of adherence with nutrition and supplement recommendations. Reinforcement of supplement recommendations and review of barriers should occur at each individual interaction. Additional serum monitoring is required if deficiency is suspected.

Supplements should be taken throughout the day as they can easily fill up a small gastric pouch or sleeve when taken all at once. Multivitamin and mineral supplements can be taken with or without food and may be crushed to increase tolerance. Enteric coated or sustained-release products should be avoided. Gastrointestinal tolerance may improve if taken with food. Drug-nutrient interactions are common with iron and calcium and may be preventable with an assessment for drug-nutrient interactions and dosing schedules.

All bariatric surgery patients should begin the recommended supplementation when they are able to tolerate solid foods (on average 2-4 weeks post surgery). For some individuals, early tolerance to tablets may be poor. This is more common in the immediate postoperative period (<14 days) or if the anastomosis is small. If the tablet or pill is <11 mm in width or length, it is usually well tolerated. [24] If there is difficulty with tolerance or the individual is concerned, alternate forms (e.g. chewable or liquid format) are available (see Table 4). Avoid "chews" or "gummy" varieties that are sticky as they may block the opening of the pouch. It is important to assess the composition of the alternate form to ensure all micronutrient needs are met.

To improve absorption of iron and calcium in a low acid environment, ferrous gluconate and calcium citrate are recommended. To improve absorption of vitamin B_{12}, forms that are not absorbed by the stomach (fast dissolve strip, sublingual or injection) are recommended. Avoid time-release and enteric coated supplements due to impaired absorption. [24]

Monitoring, Evaluation and Treatment of Vitamins and Minerals

Physical signs and symptoms of vitamin and mineral deficiencies are not specific and may not be readily observed as they present only in later stages or advancement of the deficiency [19]. Serum monitoring is recommended before surgery to assess baseline levels and should be considered a routine and essential component of care after bariatric surgery. [5, 24, 34] Biochemical monitoring is recommended to assess body stores and monitor levels with attention to iron (CBC-diff, ferritin, iron, TIBC and % sat) folic acid (folate), bone health (25-OH vitamin D, calcium and PTH) and vitamin B_{12}. Serum calcium levels should not be used to assess bone health or inform supplementation needs. Bone mineral density should be monitored every 2 years after bariatric surgery, especially in post-menopausal women. [2]

Iron

Women who have heavy menstrual periods or people with a history of anemia are at increased risk for iron deficiency. Between 9-16% of general adult women population have low iron. [24] Iron deficiency can occur in up to 49% of gastric bypass individuals. [20] Combined and malabsorptive bariatric procedures impact both the site of iron absorption (e.g. duodenum and proximal jejunum) and gastric acidity. Gastric sleeve, bypass or malabsorptive surgeries reduce the production of hydrochloric acid and therefore can impact absorption of iron. Intolerance to iron-rich foods (e.g. meat) after bariatric surgery may contribute to inadequate oral intake of this mineral. Fatigue is the most common sign and symptom, in addition to pale conjuctiva and skin tone.

Suggested Treatment

Monitor serum ferritin levels. If serum ferritin is deficient, a full iron panel is recommended (total Iron, Iron Saturation, TIBC, Hb, MCV) to assess for anemias.

Recommend a high-iron multivitamin if the current multivitamin is low in iron. For menstruating women and those at risk of anemia, target 50-100mg elemental iron/day total intake. [24] An iron supplement such as ferrous gluconate 300 mg (11% elemental = 33 mg iron), starting with one daily and increase to 3 times daily can be added as needed. Vitamin C can enhance iron absorption; taking 200mg vitamin C for 30mg elemental iron increases iron absorption by 10% [21]. A practical suggestion is to take half of a 500 mg chewable tablet with each iron pill. Some people may experience gastrointestinal side effects with iron. Taking iron supplements or high iron multivitamins (e.g. prenatal) with food or before bedtime may improve symptoms.

Continue with iron supplementation until 6 months after serum hemoglobin in normal. Re-evaluate dosing to maintain normal serum levels. For significant iron deficiencies, iron injections or transfusions may be required. Refer to physician if serum levels do not improve with oral supplementation or if individual unable to tolerate oral supplementation.

Vitamin B_{12}

Vitamin B_{12} deficiency occurs in 13% or patients seeking gastric bypass [22] and 26-70% of gastric bypass patients. [28]. It also occurs in individuals taking certain medications (e.g. acid blockers, proton-pump inhibitors, metformin). The absorption of vitamin B_{12} is complex and is impacted by combined and malabsorptive bariatric procedures. Vitamin B_{12} requires the presence of intrinsic factor for absorption in the jejunum. Reduction or impairment of the parietal cells from bariatric procedures contributes to the deficiency. Absorption is compromised due to the reduction of hydrochloric acid, impairing the release of the vitamin from protein. Signs and symptoms for low levels (serum levels < 120 pmol/L) include paresthesia, loss of cutaneous sensation and weakness. Physical signs and symptoms may not present until the deficiency is significant and may not resolve with supplementation. Excess intake of folic acid supplements (>1000 mg) may mask a B_{12} deficiency in serum but neurological symptoms will remain. [24]

Suggested Treatment

Monitor serum levels of Vitamin B_{12} (pmol/L) to assess for deficiency and effectiveness of supplementation. Ensure the multivitamin contains Vitamin B_{12}, however this will not be sufficient to prevent deficiency. [34] Vitamin B_{12} is available by tablet; however it requires gastric digestion and absorption, which is compromised after sleeve gastrectomy, gastric bypass or any malabsorptive procedures. A fast-dissolving strip (placed on the tongue) or sublingual pill is preferred over oral pills to improve absorption. American guidelines [24] recommend 350 to 500 mcg crystalline Vitamin B_{12} daily, which is not commonly available in Canada. Current recommendations for 1000 mcg are based on availability of the supplement in Canada [29]. Vitamin B_{12} injections, usually administered once per month may be required for severe deficiencies, poor adherence or response to other supplementation.

Vitamin D

Individuals with bariatric surgical procedures may have reduced vitamin and mineral intake due to low calorie diet, food intolerances and limited intake secondary to small pouch volume and narrow stoma. Although gastric bypass does not impact absorption in the jejunum and ileum, fat soluble vitamins may not optimally mix with bile salts. [23] The relationship between requirements, vitamin D status, supplementation and changes with weight loss or bariatric surgery still needs to be determined. Although some bariatric surgeries do not directly impair the digestion or absorption of vitamin D, calcium is impacted and deficiencies can persist. Deficiencies were detected in over 40% of gastric bypass patients taking a recommended dose of 1500mg calcium and 800 IU vitamin D in one study. Treatment with high dose therapy and daily supplementation was shown to safely correct low serum values after bariatric surgery [24]. Close monitoring after bariatric surgery is warranted. Refer to Chapter 3 for more information on Vitamin D.

Thiamin

Incidence of thiamin deficiency is rare but it can occur in early post operative individuals with protracted vomiting, or late (>1 year post op) in association with alcohol abuse, eating disorders or thiamin-deficient diet. Neurological complications can present due to inadequate thiamin. Signs and symptoms may include changes in gait, leg neuropathy, changes in eye movement (e.g. Wernickes, beriberi, post-operative polyneuropathy or APGARS- acute post - gastric reduction surgery). Persistent vomiting and inadequate intake can deplete body stores in a few weeks or less (average 30 mg with a half life of 9-18 days). Deficiency can occur with intakes of <0. 3mg per 1000 kcal per day (average intake adults is 2 mg per day) [27]. Serum markers respond to supplementation, but are a poor indicator of body stores. [24]

Suggested Treatment

Ensure multivitamin has 100% DRI for thiamine (1.1 mg women, 1.2 mg men) [27]. If symptoms of protracted vomiting are present, start thiamine 100 mg/day tablet orally if possible. [5, 6] Refer to a physician if signs and symptoms do not improve with oral supplementation or if individual unable to tolerate oral supplementation. If neurological symptoms are present, send the patient to the emergency department as IV therapy is required.

Nutrtion Monitoring and Evaluation after Bariatric Surgery

Based on a comprehensive nutrition assessment and information gathered as part of follow up care, the registered dietitian can assist the team with overall treatment plans. Monitoring and evaluation is a process of reviewing the patient progress and relevant data to compare with the intervention plan. Adjustments or modifications to the care plan are made with attention give to identifying and managing barriers that are preventing the patient from reaching identified goals.

Goals of treatment are determined collaboratively with the patient and the team. Outcomes are defined for each goal, based on the patient and comparative standards. To achieve the goals and outcomes, specific interventions are determined. [3] The nutrition care plan is individualized based upon patient history, surgery type, nutritional status and patient goals. A summary of key components and outcome indicators to be assessed at follow up visits after bariatric surgery is provided below.

Key Components	Outcome Indicators [25]
• Activity level • Adequacy of protein intake, evaluation when to discontinue protein supplement • Adequacy of fluid intake, fluid choices (carbonation, calorie intake), thirst • Advancement of fluid diet to solid foods • Blood work • Changes in medication or health status • Changes to taste preferences • Eating behaviours (e.g. rate/pace, meal frequency, negative self talk/irrational thoughts) • Eating environment • Food intolerances • Gastrointestinal symptoms (e.g. heartburn, emesis, gas/bloating, bowel function) • Hunger, appetite and satiety • Multivitamin and mineral supplement tolerance and intake • Self monitoring • Separation of liquids from solids • Signs and symptoms of dumping syndrome for gastric bypass • Swallowing difficulty • Volume of solid food tolerated at a meal or snack • Weight change	• Ability to use self-monitoring tools • Achieve and maintain normal serum values (multivitamins, glycemic and lipid indices) • Applies self management skills to chronic condition • Demonstrates problem solving skills as applied to food intolerances • Meeting protein requirements as evidenced by wound healing, lack of infection • Portion control • Prevention of weight re-gain • Reduction or elimination of gastrointestinal symptoms • Selection of foods and fluids consistent with recommendations • Takes multivitamin and mineral supplements as recommended • Weight loss consistent with guidelines for post operative procedure and time frame

Table 5. Factors contributing to weight re-gain after bariatric surgery [33, 4, 5]

Nutrition
• Increased caloric intake • Selection of calorie-dense foods • Increased frequency of eating: 6 or more times per day, grazing pattern of intake • Consumption of caloric beverages leading to intake above total daily calorie goal • Consumption of carbonated beverages – may contribute to increased compliance of the pouch (e.g. "pouch stretch")

- Consuming liquids within 30 minutes of a solid meal or snack, increasing total intake of solid food
- Rate of eating is too slow (grazing pattern, over 30 minutes for a meal)
- Adaptation to feelings of fullness/satiety over time; able to eat increased portion of food

Activity

- Increase in sedentary behaviour
- Decrease or discontinuation of activity
- Decreased energy expenditure (e.g. injury or illness)

Behaviour and Self Monitoring

- Decrease or discontinuation of self monitoring
- Changes to physical or mental health (e.g. depression) impacting lifestyle behaviours

Medical or Surgical

- Decreased metabolic rate: due to advancing age, decreased muscle mass, medication, disease, endocrine factors
- Medication side effects
- New diagnosis or worsening of co-morbid condition impacting lifestyle behaviours
- Surgical/Technical problems (e.g. leak of saline from appliance [LAGB], Gastro-gastric fistula [RYGB])

Weight

Weight status is an important clinical outcome and should be monitored routinely by the patient (e.g. once per week) and at each visit with their health care provider. Comparative standards for weight outcomes after bariatric surgery are variable and include to achieve and sustain 1) a 50% loss of excess weight, 2) a loss of 20-30% of total weight 3) BMI < 35 kg/m^2 [36, 4, 1]

Inadequate weight loss (<30 % excess weight loss) after a procedure may be an indication of surgical or technical failure (e.g. loss of integrity of gastric pouch), lack of proper adjustment to the LAGB, maladaptive eating behaviours or psychological complications (e.g. depression, anxiety). Excessive weight loss (>80% excess weight loss) may indicate protein/calorie malnutrition, excessive restriction of intake, excessive exercise or unintentional weight loss due to other reasons (e.g. obstructions, cancer). Investigations and referral to the appropriate health care provider are recommended. [4, 26]

There is a normal adaptation of the body after significant weight loss to achieve a stable weight. It is expected to see some weight re-gain after weight loss. With significant weight loss, there is often a significant loss in muscle mass. With activity and nutrition, a small increase in muscle mass is achievable and may result in a positive change in body composition and some weight re-gain. However, some people who have bariatric surgery may experience significant weight re-gain. Weight regain may be 20-25% of the lost weight over a 10 year period after surgery. [27] In one study, gastric bypass patients with a presurgery BMI > 50 kg/m^2 lost weight faster and re-gained more rapidly than patients with BMI <50 kg/m^2. [28] There are several factors that may contribute to weight re-gain (see Table 5). Routine monitoring of weight can identify weight gain trends and target earlier intervention. Reassessment by the bariatric team may be recommended.

Complications after Bariatric Surgery- Nutrition Implications

Bariatric surgical complication rates are well documented and reviewed in the literature. This section provides a brief summary of possible post surgical complications that have nutritional impact. Signs and symptoms of possible complications should be evaluated at follow up visits. Referral to a physician, bariatric surgeon, registered dietitian or multidisciplinary bariatric team may be warranted.

All procedures

Nausea, emesis or vomiting can be improved for most individuals with education regarding food selection and eating behaviour. Individuals with protracted vomiting should be assessed for strictures, obstructions, a LAGB that is too tight or differential diagnosis (e.g. pregnancy). Individuals with persistent or protracted vomiting should be screened for thiamine deficiency and supplemented if neurological symptoms present. [2, 5, 6]

Small bowel obstruction may present as abdominal bloating, cramping, pain and nausea to severe pain and emesis. [29] It may be due to adhesions, internal hernias or severe constipation. Increased dietary fibre is not recommended at this time.

Ulcers of the stomach or anastomosis (ie. marginal ulcers) may present as upper epigastric pain and/or burning that can radiate to the back, with symptoms of nausea, vomiting and food intolerances. Iron deficiency anemia is commonly associated with chronic ulcers. [30] Monitoring serum ferritin and iron levels is important.

Excess or loose skin is a common, unwanted side effect of significant weight loss. Mobility and self care may be impaired. Infection and ulcerations may develop, warranting nutrition intervention for wound healing.

Referral to physician or occupational/physical therapist for skin care, adaptive aids, abdominal binders or other treatment is recommended. Assessment by a plastic surgeon may be required.

Restrictive Procedures

Erosion or slippage of the band may occur. Individuals who had a LAGB or VBG may present with symptoms of dysphagia, nausea, vomiting, inability to tolerate solid food, abdominal pain or discomfort, or possible excessive weight loss. Referral to a bariatric surgeon is recommended as repositioning, replacement or removal of the band may be required. An assessment by a registered dietitian is recommended to ensure fluid and nutrition requirements are met and to determine if texture modification is required.

Leakages from port or band tubing (LAGB):[16] Individuals report feeling fullness or satiety initially after a fill, but complete loss of this sensation and significant increase in volume of solid food tolerated occurs within a few days. Weight re-gain or poor weight loss outcome may occur.

Combined Procedures

Anastomotic stricture may occur during healing as scar tissue develops. Strictures may be suspected if a recent surgical patient (e.g. RYGB) had previously been tolerating oral intake, but now reports consistent and progressive nausea and vomiting with solid foods, and is only able to tolerate small amounts of liquids at a time. Reassessment by a bariatric surgeon is recommended. The registered dietitian should assist the individual with meeting nutrition requirements and symptom management until assessed by a bariatric surgeon.

Gastro-gastric fistula may develop due to failure or incomplete staple partition of the pouch [1] Individuals may present with tolerance of high volume of solid food, lack of restriction, lack of satiety, tolerance to textures commonly difficult after bariatric procedures (sticky, doughy, stringy, tough) and either weight re-gain or poor weight loss outcome. Referral to a bariatric surgeon is recommended for assessment and possible surgical repair.

Revisional Surgery [12]

Nutrition recommendations for revisional surgery should be consistent with the guidelines for the second surgery (e.g. gastric bypass as opposed to the original gastric band) and meet requirements for other co-morbid conditions. Nutrition assessment should include evaluation for malnutrition including vitamin and mineral deficiencies.

Dumping Syndrome

Dumping syndrome is identified as a cluster of symptoms that can develop after gastric or intestinal surgery. The incidence varies from 1% to 75% [31] with an average of about 35%. [32] Dumping syndrome does not present in individuals with restrictive bariatric surgeries such as vertical banded gastroplasty, adjustable gastric band, sleeve gastrectomy or intragastric balloons. [33] The incidence of dumping syndrome after gastric bypass is as high as 75% in the early post-operative period, with a complete resolution in the majority of individuals over 15 to 18 months from surgery." [20]

Symptoms start to occur after food or beverage ingestion, presenting as early as 30 minutes (75% of individuals) or as late as 1 to 3 hours after consumption (25% of individuals). [34]

Most individuals with early dumping have both gastrointestinal (GI) and vasomotor symptoms, whereas late dumping is mostly associated with vasomotor symptoms. [35] Early dumping is due to the rapid transit of hyperosmolar particles into the intestinal lumen causing a fluid shift, increased bowel contractility and rapid small intestine distention. GI symptoms include nausea, cramping, early satiety and diarrhea.

Symptoms consistent with late-onset dumping are due to a hyperinsulinemic response resulting in reactive hypoglycemia. Vasomotor symptoms include sweating, flushing, anxiety or nervousness, increased heart rate, dizziness and an intense need to lie down.

Table 6. Nutrition Recommendations for Dumping Syndrome

	Choose	Limit
Vegetables and fruit	• All fresh and frozen vegetables • All fresh, frozen and unsweetened canned fruit • 100 % unsweetened vegetable juice	• Dried fruits, candied fruit and fruit frozen or canned in syrup • 100 % pure fruit juice (limit to ½ cup or 125 mL per day)
Grain products	• Unsweetened grains and bread products	• Sweetened cereals, sweetened baked breads like donuts, cinnamon buns and sweet rolls
Milk and alternatives	• Milk, fortified unflavoured soy milk, cream soups, artificially sweetened pudding and yogurt, cottage cheese and other cheeses	• Hot chocolate mix, chocolate milk, ice cream, frozen yogurt, milkshakes, custard, pudding, yogurt sweetened with sugar and flavoured soy milk
Meats and alternatives	• Meats, poultry, fish, seafood, eggs, nuts, peas, beans, lentils and tofu	• None
Liquids and beverages	• Water, diet pop, sugar-free and artificially sweetened beverages • Tea and coffee without sugar • Note: See list of artificial sweeteners below	• Regular pop, sugar-sweetened drink crystals, fruit drinks, fruit punches, iced tea, tea and coffee sweetened with sugar, flavoured syrup for hot or cold beverages and frozen slush drinks, liqueurs or alcohol with sweet mixes
Sweets and desserts	• Foods prepared with artificial sweeteners; diet jam and diet gelatin like sugar-free Jell-O®	• Cakes, pies, cookies, sherbet, regular gelatin, syrup, sugar, brown sugar, licorice, honey, candies, chocolate, molasses, sweet buns and rolls
Condiments	• Soy sauce, lemon juice, vinegar, salsa, unsweetened condiments and salad dressings	• Sauces with sugar like ketchup, BBQ sauce, sweet and sour sauce, jellies, jams, sweetened salad dressings, relish, sweet pickles and teriyaki sauces
Sugars and sweeteners	• Products with artificial sweeteners like Nutrasweet®, Equal®, aspartame, Splenda®, sucralose, Sweet and Low® and Acesulfame potassium (Ace-K)	• Sugars: glucose, sucrose, fructose, lactose, dextrose, honey, molasses, maltose, syrups, fruit juice concentrate • Sugar alcohols: sorbitol, mannitol, maltitol, isomalt and xylitol
Fats, oils and high fat foods	• Fats, oils and high fat foods such as deep fried foods or gravies do not cause dumping syndrome. However, some people may experience an increase in bowel movements with these foods.	

Approximately 1 to 5% of GI surgery individuals [20] and 10 to 15% [36] of gastric bypass individuals will have severe symptoms that continue despite changes to the diet. [18] Individuals with hyperinsulinemic hypoglycemia that do not improve, especially with late dumping, should be assessed by a physician as pharmacologic therapy or surgical treatment may be required. [22, 37] Individuals with severe dumping syndrome can present with significant weight loss and malnutrition. [18] The weight loss may easily be misinterpreted as an intended and appropriate outcome of bariatric surgery. Regular patient follow-up including detailed intake, symptom and weight history will help to identify and manage dumping syndrome. [18]

Nutrition Recommendations for Dumping Syndrome [20] (See Table 6)

Food intake should be divided into small meals and snacks taken 4 to 6 times throughout the day. Meals that include the addition of fibre, are low to moderate fat and adequate protein can assist with hypoglycaemia, rapid absorption and transit time. Psyllium is hydrophilic and can increase fecal water holding capacity [23] and is effective for both diarrhea and constipation symptoms. Complex carbohydrates and high-fibre foods should be included regularly in the diet. Restrictions for meat and meat-alternative foods or fats are not required so can be used to replace calories from carbohydrates to meet daily energy requirements. [18] Foods high in sugar should be limited or avoided. Some individuals may misuse sugars to induce dumping syndrome to address constipation issues or as an attempt to promote weight loss. Detailed symptom and food/nutrient intake history helps tp identify this concern and appropriate education and support can be provided.

Fluid intake should be avoided during and at least 30 minutes before and after eating solid foods. Only small amounts of fluid (up to 125 ml) should be consumed at a time. Fluids should be sipped slowly. If rapid emptying of the stomach or gastric pouch is a concern, lying down for 30 minutes after eating can assist to delay gastric emptying and reduce the risk of syncope. However, if heartburn is present, it is not recommended to lie down after eating as this may worsen the symptoms.

Tolerance to milk and milk products is variable after bariatric surgery. Temporary lactose intolerance may develop after surgery, illness or if diarrhea is frequent. Short-term restriction of lactose may be needed until GI symptoms improve. Lactose may be reintroduced gradually once symptoms improve.

Conclusion

Nutrition care after bariatric surgery can help maintain or improve nutritional status, minimize nutrition-related complications and assist patients to develop lifestyle behaviours to improve their weight and health. Monitoring and evaluation after bariatric surgery is recommended beyond the immediate post-operative period as nutritional deficiencies and complications may present at a later stage. Vitamin and mineral supplementation after bariatric surgery is required and should be continued long term.

To achieve and maintain health and weight outcomes, significant lifestyle changes are required for a lifetime and include healthy eating habits, regular physical activity, self-monitoring and stress management. Prevention of weight re-gain is an important clinical outcome and requires ongoing monitoring, nutrition intervention, activity and behaviour modification.

Acknowledgments

The authors wish to acknowledge Nutrition Services, Alberta Health Service for their permission to use the Nutrition Practice Guidelines for Registered Dietitians for Adult Bariatric Care and the contributions and expertise of the AHS Registered Dietitians and members of the Adult Bariatric Care Nutrition Working Group.

References

[1] Lau DCW, Douketis JD, Morrison KM, Hramiak IM, Sharma AM, Ur E. for the Obesity Canada Clinical Practice Guidelines Expert Panel. 2006 Canadian clinical practice guidelines on the management and prevention of obesity in adults and children. *CMAJ* 2007;176(8):S1-13. Available from: URL: http://www.cmaj.ca/cgi/reprint/176/8/S1.

[2] Gastrointestinal surgery for severe obesity. National Institutes of Health consensus development conference statement. *Am. J. Clin. Nutr.* 1992;55 Suppl 2:615S-9S.

[3] Douketis JD, Macie C, Thabane L, Williamson DF. Systematic review of long term weight loss studies in obese adults: clinical significance and applicability to clinical practice. *Int. J. Obes.* 2005;29:1153-67.

[4] Mechanick JI, Kushner RF, Sugerman HJ, Gonzalez-Campoy M, Collazo-Clavell ML, Guven S, et al. AACE/TOS/ASMBS Guidelines. American Association of Clinical Endocrinologists, The Obesity Society, and American Society for Metabolic and Bariatric Surgery medical guidelines for the clinical practice for the perioperative nutritional, metabolic and nonsurgical support of the bariatric surgery individual. *Surg. Obes. Relat. Dis.* 2008;4:S109-84.

[5] Aills L, Blakenship J, Buffington C, Furtado M, Parrott J. American Society for Metabolic and Bariatric Surgery: ASMBS Allied Health Nutritional Guidelines for the Surgical Weight Loss Individual. *Surg. Obes. Rel. Dis.* 2008;4:S73-S108.

[6] Chapman AE, Kiroff G, Game P, Foster B, O'Brien P, Ham J. Laparoscopic adjustable gastric banding in the treatment of obesity: a systematic literature review. *Surgery* 2004;135:326-51.

[7] Stroh C, Birk D, Flade-Kuthe R, Frenken M, Herbig B, Hohne S. Bariatric Surgery Working Group. Results of sleeve gastrectomy - data from a nationwide survey on bariatric surgery in Germany. *Obes. Surg.* 2009;19(5):632-40.

[8] Tagaya N, Kasama K, Kikkawa R, Kanahira E, Umezawa A, Oshiro T et al. Experience with laparoscopic sleeve gastrectomy for morbid versus super morbid obesity. *Obes. Surg.* 2008;19(10):1371-76.

[9] Frezza EE, Reddy S, Gee LL, Wachtel MS. Complications after sleeve gastrectomy for morbid obesity. *Obes. Surg.* 2008;19(6):684-7.

[10] Bernstine H, Tzioni-Yehoshua R, Groshar D, Beglaibter N, Shikora S, Rosenthal RJ, et al. Gastric Emptying is not affected by sleeve gastrectomy-scintigraphic evaluation of gastric emptying after sleeve gastrectomy without removal of the gastric antrum. *Obes. Surg.* 2009;19:293-8.

[11] American Society for Metabolic and Bariatric Surgery. Updated Position statement on sleeve gastrectomy as a bariatric procedure. 2011. Available from: www.asmbs.org.
[12] Lim CSH, Liew V, Talbot ML, Jorgensen JO, Loi KW. Revisional Bariatric Surgery. *Obes. Surg*. 2008;19(7):827-32.
[13] Jorgensen S, Olesen M, Gudman-Hoyer E. A review of 20 years of jejuonileal bypass. *Sand. J. Gastroenterol.* 1997;32:334-9.
[14] Laverson JD. Micronutrient deficiencies after gastric bypass for morbid obesity. *Am. Surg*. 1986;52:594-8.
[15] Xanthakos SA, Inge TH. Nutritional consequences of bariatric surgery. *Curr. Opin. Clin. Nutr. Metab. Care* 2006;9:489-96.
[16] Jeffery KM, Harkins B, Cresci GA, Martindale RG. The clear liquid diet is no longer a necessity in the routine postoperative management of surgical patients. *Am. J. Surg*. 1996;62:167–70.
[17] The American Heritage Medical Dictionary. Houghton Mifflin Company, Boston MA. 2007.
[18] National Academies of Science. Dietary Reference Intakes for energy, carbohydrate, fibre, fat, fatty acids, cholesterol, protein, and amino acids. National Academies Press, Washington DC. 2005. Available from:http://www.nap.edu/catalog.php?record_id=10490.
[19] Harrison's Principles of Internal Medicine. Chapter 71: Vitamin and Trace Mineral Deficiency and Excess. 17th Edition. McGraw-Hill Medical, New York NY. 2008.
[20] Brolin RE, Gorman JH, Gorman RC, Petschenik AJ, Bradley LJ, Kenler HA et al. Are vitamin B12 and folate deficiency clinically important after Roux-en-Y gastric bypass? *J. Gastrointest. Surg*. 1998;2:436-42.
[21] Compendium of Pharmaceuticals and Specialties (CPS). The Canadian Drug Reference for Health Professionals. Canadian Pharmacists Association, 2012. Available from www.e-cps.ca or http://www.e-therapeutics.ca (Membership required).
[22] Madan AK, Orth WS, Tichansky DS, Ternovits CA. Vitamin and trace mineral levels after laparoscopic gastric bypass. *Obes. Surg*. 2006;16:603-6.
[23] Mahlay NF, Verka LG, Thomsen K, Merugu S, Salomone M. Vitamin D Status before roux-en-y and efficacy of prophylactic and therapeutic doses of vitamin D in individuals after roux-en-y gastric bypass surgery. *Obes. Surg*. 2008;19(5):590-4.
[24] Carlin AM, Rao DS, Yager KM, Parikh JN, Kapke A, Treatment of vitamin D depletion after roux- en-y-gastric bypass: a randomized prospective clinical trial. *Surg. Obes. Relat. Dis*. 2009;5(4):444-49.
[25] American Dietetic Association. ADA Pocket Guide to Bariatric Surgery. Weight Management Practice Group. American Dietetic Association. Chicago, IL 2009.
[26] Snyder B, Nguyen A, Scarbourough T, Yu S, Wilson E. Comparison of those who succeed in losing significant excessive weight after bariatric surgery and those who fail. *Surg. Endosc*. 2009;01(30).
[27] Heber D, Greenway FL, Kaplan LM, Livingston E Salvador J, Still C. Endocrine and Nutritional Management of the Post-Bariatric Surgery Patient: An Endocrine Society Clinical Practice Guideline. *J. Clin. Endocriol. Metab*. 2010;95:4823-43.
[28] Christou NV, Look D, MacLean LD. Weight gain after short- and long-limb gastric bypass in patients followed for longer than 10 years. *Ann. Surg*. 2006;24:734-40.

[29] Lanyon RI, Maxwell BM, Kraft AJ. Prediction of long-term outcome after gastric bypass surgery. *Obes. Surg.* 2008;19(4):439-45.

[30] de Jong JR, van Ramshorst B, Gooszen HG, Smout AJPM, Tiel-Van Buul MMC. Weight loss after laparoscopic adjustable gastric banding is not caused by altered gastric emptying. *Obes. Surg.* 2009;19:287-92.

[31] Radigan AE. Post-Gastrectomy: Managing the Nutrition Fall-Out. Nutrition Issues in Gastroenterology, Series #18. *Practical Gastroenterology* June 2004;63-75.

[32] Thomson ABR, Padda S, Ramirez R, Aguirre T. Dumping Syndrome. 26 Jan 2010. © eMedicine from WebMD. Available from http://emedicine.medscape.com/article/173594-overview.

[33] Decker GA, Swain JM, Crowell MD, Scolapio JS. Gastrointestinal and Nutritional Complications After Bariatric Surgery. *Am. J. Gastroenterol.* 2007;102:2571-80.

[34] Ukleja, A. Dumping syndrome: Pathophysiology and Treatment. *Nutr. Clin. Pract.* 2005;20:517-25.

[35] Dumping Syndrome. © Mayo Foundation for Medical Education and Research (MFMER) 1998-2008 Available from http://www.mayoclinic.com/health/dumping-syndrome/DS00715.

[36] Goldfine AB, Mun E, Patti ME. Hyperinsulinemic hypoglycemia following gastric bypass surgery for obesity. *Current Opinion in Endocrinology and Diabetes* 2006;13: 419-424.

[37] Fedorak RN, Borowiec AM. Symptom Control: Diarrhea. Therapeutic Choices. © Canadian Pharmacists Association 2009. Available from https://www.e-therapeutics.ca/wps.

In: The Fundamentals of Bariatric Surgery
Editors: Shahzeer Karmali and Daniel W. Birch
ISBN: 978-1-62417-732-3

Chapter 15

Biliary Complications Associated with Morbid Obesity and Obesity Reducing Surgery

Jean-Francois Ouellet and Chad G. Ball
University of Calgary, Calgary, Alberta, Canada

Introduction

Morbid obesity is a continually increasing public health concern and is linked to multisystem comorbid diseases such as biliary pathology [1, 2]. While surgery for morbid obesity has been shown to reverse many of these comorbidities [3, 4], the risk of biliary stone (cholelithiasis) formation is actually increased following weight reduction. More specifically, the incidence of gallstone formation following bariatric procedures ranges from 10% to 71% [5, 6] and is dependant on the type of surgery. This increased lithogenesis is believed to be multifactorial [5, 7, 8] (Table 1), as well as maximal during periods of rapid weight loss. Retrospective studies have identified factors such as weight loss at three months of more than 50 % excess weight [5] or excess weight loss greater than 75 % at 2 years post laparoscopic roux-en-Y gastric bypass (LRYGB) [9] as clearly predictive of biliary subsequent complications.

Table 1. Factors increasing gallbladder stone formation following bariatric surgeryref [4, 3, 9]

- Increase cholesterol saturation in bile due to cholesterol mobilization from fatty tissues
- Decreased secretion of biliary acids due to caloric restriction
- Increased mucin production
- Gallbladder hymotility due to
    - decreased cholecystokinin (hypocaloric diet, gastroduodenal exclusion)
    - injury to hepatic branch of vagus nerve

Table 2. Support for and againts routine cholecystectomy at the time of LRYGB

Positive	Negative
Increased incidence of biliary tract disease in the setting of rapid weight loss	Overestimation of patients with symptomatic gallstones following LRYGB
Low yield of pre-operative ultrasound to identify patients with cholelithiasis	Potentially increased operative time Potentially increased operative stay
Low compliance to prophylactic ursodeoxycholic acid therapy post-operatively	Alteration in port-placement
Potentially complicated cholecystectomy if required post-operatively	Difficulty performing a cholecystectomy in a morbidly obese patient
Difficulty accessing common bile duct in the setting of a Roux-en-Y configuration	Effectiveness of ursodeoxycholic acid in reducing gallstone formation post-operatively

Reports outlining the true incidence of symptomatic cholelithiasis requiring cholecystectomy after RYGB are conflicting, but range from 3% to 28% [5, 10-15]. While all clinicians believe that there is a true increased risk of symptomatic cholelithiasis following bariatric procedures, conflicting views in regards to the prevention of gallstone formation persist, especially in patients undergoing LRYGB procedure. Additionally, a recent meta-analysis of randomized controlled trials [6] has confirmed the effectiveness of ursodeoxycholic acid (UDCA) in the prevention of gallstone formation after bariatric surgery. Analyzing a total of 521 patients from 5 placebo-controlled studies, this meta-analysis shows that a daily dose of at least 500 mg is an effective prophylactic modality. Most authors in favour of this approach recommend 6 months of therapy after surgery [7, 16-17]. One drawback of this therapy however is the frequently limited compliance, , with rates ranging from 28% to 80% [14, 16-17]. Because LRYGB is currently the dominant bariatric procedure performed worldwide, this chapter will mainly focus on the role of cholecystectomy at the time of a LRYGB, as well as the management of biliary complications following LRYGB.

Role of Routine Cholecystectomy at the Time of LRYGB

Despite multiple publications, significant controversy remains as to whether prophylactic cholecystectomy is indicated at the time of LRYGB (Table 2). While all agree that patients with symptomatic cholelilithiasis should underdo cholecystectomy at the time of the LRYGB, a variety of approaches have been proposed in the absence of cholelithiasis pre-operatively, or in the setting of asymptomatic cholelilithiasis.

Management of Asymptomatic Gallstones Identical to Nonobese Patients

Despite strong criticism, some authors have suggested that asymptomatic gallstones in bariatric patients should be treated in the same manner as in the nonobese population. Swartz and Felix published their center's experience in 2005, where asymptomatic patients underwent neither preoperative screening gallbladder ultrasound (US), nor concomitant cholecystectomy at the time of their LRYGB [15]. In this series of 319 patients, only 47 (14.7%) eventually required a cholecystectomy. Of these, 93.6 % were performed laparoscopically with a complication rate of 4.4 %. As a result, they proposed an approach based on post-operative symptom occurrence only, omitting routine pre-operative US in all asymptomatic patients. It must be mentioned as a significant limitation that the majority of patients were also placed on prophylactic ursodeoxycholic acid therapy for 6 months post-operatively and that their median follow-up time was only 7.5 months.

Similarly, Patel and colleagues. presented their experience in 2006 where patients undergoing LRYGB were also not routinely screened for gallstones, nor were they treated medically on a prophylactic basis with bile salts [13]. They reported a series of 199 patients of which only 12 (6%) required cholecystectomy for gallstone-induced pathology after undergoing a LRYGB procedure (mean follow up period of 17.8 months). Laparoscopic removal was performed in almost all patients (92%). These similar results lead the authors to plead that more aggressive approaches may not be necessary.

Routine Pre-operative or Intra-operative US Screening and Cholecystectomy in All Patients with Proven Gallstones

This popular surgical approach requires evaluation of the gallbladder either pre-operatively or intra-operatively. Screening ultrasound in all patients is supported by observations that 15 to 20% of patients undergoing weight-reducing surgery have cholelithiasis on pre-operative imaging (90% asymptomatic) [18]. While some authors had previously described longer operative times and hospital stays in patients undergoing simultaneous cholecystectomy at the time of LRYGB [19], more recent series challenge this finding. More specifically, Escalona published a series of 1174 patients who underwent LRYGB where 128 patients (10.9%) had a simultaneous cholecystectomy due to cholelithiasis and/or gallbladder polyps identified on pre-operative US [18]. When comparing surgical results between the two groups (simultaneous cholecystectomy vs without cholecystectomy), operative time was slightly longer in the cholecystectomy group (21 minutes), although there was no difference in length of hospital stay, conversion rate or post-operative complications. No conversions to open surgery or post-operative complications were directly related to a cholecystectomy. It must also be noted that the patients in the cholecystectomy group were older and had a greater preoperative BMI.

Tucker et al. also published their experience with this "selective approach" to the gallbladder at the time of LRYGP [10]. At their institution, concomitant cholecystectomy was planned in all patients with US-confirmed cholelithiasis and/or a gallbladder polyp greater than 1 cm. In a cohort of more than 1700 patients, 12 % (205 patients) met the trigger to undergo concomitant cholecystectomy. Of these, 123 patients eventually underwent a cholecystectomy. Again, a mild increase in the mean operative time (18 minutes) was noted in the cholecystectomy group with no impact on hospital length of stay. One patient did present with a bile leak post-cholecystectomy managed by laparoscopic transgastrostomy endoscopic retrograde cholangiopancreatocgraphy. Interestingly, 68 patients did not undergo cholecystectomy despite preoperative US detected cholelithiasis. Subsequent cholecystectomy was required in 17.6 % of these patients. All were performed laparoscopically, with one patient requiring laparoscopic common bile duct exploration. Of the patients who had an initial normal pre-operative US, 6 % eventually developed symptomatic cholelithiasis (mean follow-up 30.5 months) requiring intervention.

Both of these authors, among many others, advocate for routine concomitant cholecystectomy at the time of LRYGB for all patients with proven gallbladder disease pre-operatively. This is supported by excellent safety profiles, a small increase in operative time, and no or minimal associated morbidity. This approach reduces the risk of post-operative gallbladder-related pathologies requiring reoperation and readmission.

Routine Prophylactic Cholecystectomy at the Time of Surgery

Several groups in the era of open gastric bypass have advocated for prophylactic cholecystectomy even in the absence of abnormal findings on pre-operative ultrasound [10, 20-21]. Reports of high incidence (60-95%) of pathologic gallbladders identified at the time of surgery despite negative preoperative US remains the dominant justification for this prophylactic approach [20, 21]. Even in the setting of open surgery, some authors would argue against prophylactic cholecystectomy in the absence of palpable gallstones, quoting a low incidence of symptomatic gallstones following gastric bypass. More directly, a significant number of patients would undergo unnecessary cholecystectomies [22]. The advent of LRYGB procedures has added more controversy to this topic as some argue that a laparoscopic cholecystectomy can be difficult in the setting of morbid obesity, and therefore supporting avoidance of this prophylactic approach in the absence of proven cholelithisasis.

The role of prophylactic cholecystectomy in the setting of LRYGB remains highly controversial and debated in the recent literature where pre-operative factors that can help identify patients at the highest risk of developing post-operative symptomatic cholelithiasis remain unclear. D'Hondt et al. failed to identify any pre-operative factors that could predict the development of symptomatic gallbladder stones following LRYGB [9]. In their series of 645 patients, 6.9 % developed symptomatic gallstones (median follow-up 51 months) post-LRYBG. The sole significant independent predictor of delayed cholecystectomy after LRYGB was weight loss at 3 months greater than 50 % of excess weight. As a result, they still recommended a conservative approach and do not advocate for prophylactic cholecystectomy.

Other authors argue that routine cholecystectomy in the setting of LRYGB can be viewed as an acceptable form of prophylaxis against future gallstone formation. Nougou and Suter [8], published their experience with a general policy to offer cholecystectomy at the time of LRYGB to all patients, regardless of pre-operative US findings, providing it could be done safely. They present a series of 714 LRYGB patients where 655 (91.7%) underwent simultaneous cholecystectomy. 576 (80.1%) had a normal pre-operative US. No differences in hospital stay and no cholecystectomy related complications were noted. As previously published, a high percentage of the gallbladders removed had abnormal histopathologic features, in addition to a false negative rate of pre-operative US approximating 3.9 % for gallstones. As a result, prophylactic cholecystectomy would be an acceptable option for post-LRYGB gallstone prophylaxis.

In the first published comparative cohort study, Tarantino et al. compared two cohorts of patients undergoing LRYGB: patients who underwent a cholecystectomy only if pre-operative US confirmed cholelithiasis, sludge or polyps, and patients who received routine cholecystectomy at the time of surgery [5]. At a median follow-up of 3.1 years, 18.6 % of the patients that did not undergo cholecystectomy during their LRYGB developed symptomatic cholelithiasis requiring surgical intervention. Of note, no patients received prophylactic ursodeoxycholic acid therapy post-operatively. Their biliary complication free survival rate after LRYGB in the setting of selective cholecystectomy was 85.5 % at 2 years, 84.3 % at 3 years, 81.3 % at 4 years and 77.4 % at 5 years. Their number needed to treat with prophylactic cholecystectomy was seven after 2 years post-operatively and 4 at 5 years. No differences in the operative outcomes, hospital stay, or excess weight loss at 2 years were noted between each cohort. Additionally, no complications were directly linked to the cholecystectomy itself. Based on their findings, they conclude that prophylactic cholecystectomy should be considered in all LRYGB procedures.

In summary, despite the fact that morbid obesity and rapid weight loss following LRYGBP are known risk factors for cholelithisasis and gallbladder complications, the optimal approach to preventing the development of gallstones complications following surgery is still debated. While level one data exists supporting the use of ursodeoxycholic acid therapy for 6 months post-operatively, the compliance rate associated with this regimen generates contemplation that a more aggressive approach to the gallbladder may be best. Selective cholecystectomy in patients with preoperative US proven cholelithiasis is favoured by many centers but does not eliminate the risk of developing gallstones post-operatively or the risk of false negative US. Finally, some centers continue to offer routine cholecystectomy in all patients undergoing LRYGPB with results showing that this procedure is safe with no added morbidity, and therefore a reduction in the risk of developing gallbladder stones and their complications. To quote Nougou and Suter [8]: "*only a large randomized trial comparing cholecystectomy at the time of LRYGP with a 6 month pharmacological prevention will answer the question as to which method is superior for gallstone prophylaxis after LRYGP.*"

Management of Biliary Complications Following RYGB

Following RYGBP, access to the biliary tree by endoscopic retrograde cholangiopancreatography (ERCP) poses a particular challenge to physicians due to the Roux-en-Y configuration and creation of the gastric pouch disconnected from the gastric remnant. This Roux-en-Y anatomy is even more challenging in the setting of RYGBP with longer Roux-limbs usually created for the purpose of weight loss compared to the standard hepatico-jejunostomy. This has been one of the dominant arguments of the proponents for prophylactic cholecystectomy. While cholecystectomy could prevent most potential post-operative gallstone complications, patients still remain at risk for other pancreato-biliary conditions requiring access to the biliary tree such as sphincter of Oddi dysfunction (SOD), pancreatitis, retained or primary choledocolithiasis and other conditions such as upper gastrointestinal bleeds (i.e.requiring access to the duodenum).

While laparoscopic or open common bile duct exploration through the transcystic route or choledochotomy remain established modalities for clearance of common bile duct stones, other less invasive techniques have been described for patients with Roux-Y configurations, when standard ERCP is impossible due to the loss of direct access to the duodenum:

Retrograde Trans-oral Endoscopy

Although high failure rates of access to the ampulla using standard side-view duodenoscopy in the setting of Roux-Y anatomy have been reported [23-24], the advent of double-balloon endoscopy has made trans-oral ERCP in post-RYGBP patients feasible. An increasing number of centers have reported their experience with this novel technique, with some reaching the bilio-pancreatic limb in 90 % of cases and completing successful ERCP in 80 % of patients [23]. These numbers must be interpreted with caution, since most publications are dominated by patients with standard hepatico-jejunostomy (i.e. shorter Roux-limbs than patients with RYGB). Despite the degree of difficulty, this procedure has also been reported in patients with prior RYGB. Emmet and Mallat published their experience with double-balloon ERCP in the setting of Roux-en-Y anatomy in 14 patients, 6 of whom had prior RYGBP [25]. In these six patients, the ampulla was reached in 100% of cases and adequate cannulation of the ampulla achieved in 88 % of patients.

It must be remembered that experienced endoscopists working in high volume centers performed these procedures and that potential difficulties are numerous: difficulty navigating through the long Roux-limb; difficulty identifying the afferent biliary-limb due to its acute angle; difficulty cannulating the ampulla due to retrograde access; limited instrumentation due to length of scopes [26].

Laparoscopic/Open Assisted Transgastric ERCP

This novel technique is particularly appealing in the setting of prior RYGBP. Performed in the operating room under general anesthesia, it mainly consists of creating an access to the gastric remnant for insertion of the duodenoscope. Most authors describe placing a pursestring suture on the gastric remnant, creating a small gastrotomy and inserting a 15 mm port directly into the stomach which will accept the side-view duodenoscope [26-30]. The ERCP can then be performed in the usual antegrade fashion through the gastric remnant and duodenum. Due to the fact that this procedure requires laparoscopic (or open) access to the abdominal cavity, another potential advantage is that a full exploration of the abdomen is possible (i.e. permits identification of other potential causes of abdominal pain (e.g. internal hernias).

Gutierrez et al. have published the most extensive experience with this technique in patients requiring ERCP or evaluation of their duodenum post-RYGBP [30] (32 procedures). All underwent successful trans-gastric approaches either laparoscopically (84.4%) or open (15.6%). The indications included: SOD (13), pancreatitis (6), choledocholithiasis (5), cholangitis (3), pancreatic mass evaluation (2), upper gastro-intestinal bleed (2) and cystic duct leak (1). For cases requiring ERCP, successful cannulation of the pancreatico-biliary tree was performed in all patients. In addition, unsuspected internal hernias were identified in one third of cases. Three patients required surgical reexploration: 1 for pancreatitis initially thought to be peritonitis and 2 for leaks at the gastrostomy site. Other groups have published smaller series with similar results and low rates of complications [26-29]. Some also report a similar approach with trans-enteric access directly at the bilio-pancreatic limb [28].

Percutaneous Transgastric ERCP

Similar to the previous technique, this approach implies percutaneous placement of a gastrostomy tube in the gastric remnant followed by serial dilatation of the tract every 2-3 weeks until it achieves a sufficient size to accept an endoscope. While this approach might appear less invasive, serial dilatations of the tract makes it less appealing, especially in settings where urgent access to the biliary tree is required.

Percutaneous Transhepatic Instrumentation of Common Bile Duct

Multiple case series of common bile duct stones management using percutaneous techniques have been described since the early 1980's [31, 32]. Burhenne's stone extraction technique with steerable baskets passed through T-tubes is the most commonly quoted approach [33]. It the absence of a T-tube, others have used this technique using a transhepatic biliary percutaneous approach and extraction of stones using *Dorma baskets* through the dilated tract. Due to limitations in the size of the tract provided by this percutaneous transhepatic approach compared to T-tubes, another interesting published alternative involves dilatation of the ampulla using angioplasty catheters placed through a transhepatic biliary drain and pushing common bile duct stones with occlusion balloons through the ampulla. This method has been shown to be successful in the majority of cases with minimal morbity. In a series of 100 cases, García-Vila et al [34] reported a success rate of 95 % with complete clearance of ductal stones with a complication rate of 5 % (1 case of pancreatitis, 4 cases of hemobilia with one requiring surgical intervention).

Case reports of percutaneous choledocoscopy and sphincterotomy through transhepatic biliary drains have also been published. Initially described by Niura et al. in 1982 [35-36], others have modified this technique over time. For example, Itoi et al. described 3 successful cases of an endoscopic sphincterotomy using a percutaneous transhepatic cholangioscope in patients with endoscopically inaccessible papilla due to prior gastric surgery [35]. Case reports of transhepatic choledocoscopy and balloon sphincteroplasty in post-LRYGBP have also been reported [36].

In summary, despite the fact that conventional ERCP is impossible in patients with prior RYGBP, options are available before considering surgical exploration of the common bile duct in the instance of post-operative biliary complications. It should be emphasized that these techniques require significant expertise in the management of patients with Roux-en-Y anatomy and a multidisciplinary team including surgeons with experience in modern bariatric surgery, dedicated interventional gastroenterologist and interventional radiologist is the key. The best approach remains to be defined but should take into consideration the local expertise available, the acuity of symptoms, the surgical risk of the patient, the potential need for multiple ERCP (where a permanent gastrostomy through the gastric remnant should be considered), the location of the biliary disorder (intra-hepatic vs extra-hepatic) and finally the length of the Roux-limb [23].

References

[1] Ogden CL, Carroll MD, Curtin LR et al., Prevalence of overweight and obesity in the United States. *JAMA*. 295: 13; 1549-1555.

[2] Must A, Spadano J, Coakley EH et al., The disease burden associated with overweight and obesity. *JAMA* 1999; 282: 16; 1523-1529.

[3] Buchwald H, Avidor Y, Braunwald E et al., Bariatric surgery: a systematic review and meta-analyses. *JAMA* 2004; 292: 14; 1724-1737.

[4] Maggard MA, Shugarman LR, Suttorp M et al., Meta-analysis: surgical treatment of obesity. *Ann. Intern. Med*. 2005; 142: 7; 547-559.

[5] Tarantino I, Warschkow R, Steffen T et al., Is Routine Cholecystectomy Justified in Severely Obese Patients Undergoing a Laparoscopic Roux-en-Y Gastric Bypass Procedure? A Comparative Cohort Study. *Obes. Surg*. 2011; 21: 12; 1870-1878.

[6] Manley C. Uy, Marilyn C. T, Wendell Z. E et al., Ursodeoxycholic Acid in the Prevention of Gallstone Formation after Bariatric Surgery: A Meta-analysis. *Obes. Surg*. 2008; 18: 12; 1532-1538.

[7] Desbeaux A, Hec F, Andrieux S et al., Risk of biliary complications in bariatric surgery. *Journal of Visceral Surgery* 2010; 147: 4; e217-e220.

[8] Nougou A, Suter M. Almost Routine Prophylactic Cholecystectomy During Laparoscopic Gastric Bypass is Safe. *Obes. Surg*. 2008; 18: 5; 535-539.

[9] D'Hondt M., Sergeant G., Deylgat B et al., Prophylactic Cholecystectomy, a Mandatory Step in Morbidly Obese Patients Undergoing Laparoscopic Roux-en-Y Gastric Bypass ? *J. Gastrointest. Surg*. 2011; 15: 9; 1532-1536.

[10] Tucker ON, Fajnwaks P, Szomstein S et al., Is concomitant cholecystectomy necessary in obese patients undergoing laparoscopic gastric bypass surgery? *Surg. Endosc*. 2008; 22: 11; 2450-2454.

[11] Shiffman ML, Sugerman HJ, Kellum JM et al., Gallstone formation after rapid weight loss: a prospective study in patients undergoing gastric bypass surgery for treatment of morbid obesity. *Am. J. Gastroenterol*. 1991; 86: 8; 1000-1005.

[12] Taylor J, Leitman IM, Horowitz M et al., Is routine cholecystectomy necessary at the time of Roux-en-Y gastric bypass? *Obes. Surg*. 2006; 16: 6; 179-761.

[13] Patel KR, White SC, Teririan T et al., Gallbladder management during laparoscopic Roux-en-Y gastric bypass surgery: routine preoperative screening for gallstones and postoperative medical treatment are not necessary. *Am. Surg*. 2006; 72: 10; 857-861.

[14] Wudel Jr LJ, Wright JK, Debelak JP et al., Prevention of gallstone formation in morbidly obese patients undergoing rapid weight loss: results of a randomized controlled pilot study. *J. Surg. Res*. 2002; 102: 1; 50-56.

[15] Swartz D, Felix E, Elective cholecystectomy after Roux-en-Y gastric bypass: why should asymptomatic gallstones be treated differently in morbidly obese patients? *Surg. Obes. Relat. Dis*. 2005; 1: 6; 555-560.

[16] Sugerman HJ, Brewer WH, Shiffman ML et al., A Multicenter placebo-controlled, randomized, double-blind prospective trial of prophylactic ursodiol for prevention of gallstone formation following gastric-bypass-induced rapid weight loss. *Am. J. Surg.* 1995; 169: 1; 91-96.

[17] Miller K, Hell E, Lang B et al., Gallstone formation prophylaxis after gastric restrictive procedure for weight loss – A randomized double-blind placebo-controlled trial. *Ann. Surg.* 2003; 238: 5; 697-702.

[18] Escalona A, Boza C, Munoz R et al., Routine Preoperative Ultrasonography and Selective Cholecystectomy in Laparoscopic Roux-en-Y Gastric Bypass. Why Not? *Obes. Surg.* 2008; 18: 1; 47-51.

[19] Hamad GG, Ikramuddin S, Gourash WF et al., Elective cholecystectomy during laparoscopic Roux-en-Y gastric bypass: is it worth the wait? *Obes. Surg.* 2003; 13: 1; 76-81.

[20] Fobi M, Lee H, Igwe D et al., Prophylactic cholecystectomy with gastric bypass operation: incidence of gallbladder disease. *Obes. Surg.* 2002; 12: ; 350-353.

[21] Liem RK, Niloff PH, Prophylactic cholecystectomy with open gastric bypass operation. *Obes. Surg.* 2004; 14: 6; 763-765.

[22] Caruana JA, McCabe MN, Smith AD et al., Incidence of symptomatic gallstones after gastric bypass: is prophylactic treatment really necessary? *Surg. Obes. Relat. Dis.* 2005; 1: 6; 564-577.

[23] Khashab M, Okolo III P. Accessing the Pancreatobiliary Limb and ERCP in the Bariatric Patient. *Gastrointest. Endoscopy Clin. N. Am.* 2011; 2: 305-313.

[24] Lopes T, Wilcox C, Endoscopic Retrograde Cholangiopancreatography in Patients with Roux-en-Y Anatomy. *Gastroenterol. Clin. N. Am.* 2010; 39; 99–107.

[25] Emmett DS, Mallat DB. Double-balloon ERCP in patients who have undergone Roux-en-Y surgery: a case series. *Gastrointest. Endosc.* 2007; 66: 5; 1038–41.

[26] Patel J, Patel N, Shinde T et al., Endoscopic Retrograde Cholangiopanereatography after Laparoscopic Roux-en-Y Gastric Bypass: A Case Series and Review of the Literature. *Am. Surg.* 2008; 74: 8; 689-694.

[27] Ceppa F, Gagne D, Papasavas P et al., Laparoscopic transgastric endoscopy after Roux-en-Y gastric bypass. *Surg. Obes. Relat. Dis.* 2007; 3: 21-24.

[28] Lopes T, Clements R, Wilcox C. Laparoscopy-assisted ERCP: experience of a high-volume bariatric surgery center (with video). *Gastrointestinal Endoscopy* 2009; 70: 6; 1254-1259.

[29] Saleem A, Levy M, Peterson B et al., Laparoscopic Assisted ERCP in Roux-en-Y Gastric Bypass (RYGB) Surgery Patients. *J. Gastrointest. Surg.* 2012; 16: 203-208.

[30] Gutierrez J, Lederer H, Krook J. Surgical Gastrostomy for Pancreatobiliary and Duodenal Access Following Roux en Y Gastric Bypass. *J. Gastrointest. Surg.* 2009; 13: 12; 2170-2175.

[31] Ilgit W, Gurel K, Onal B. Percutaneous management of bile duct stones, *European Journal of Radiology* 2002: 43; 237-245.

[32] Geisinger M, Owens D, Meaney T. Radiology methods of bile duct stone extraction. *AJR* 1989; 158: 222-227.

[33] Burhenne HJ. Nonoperative retained biliary tract stone extrac tion: a new roentgenologic technique. *Am. J. Roentgenol.* 1973;117:388 – 99.

[34] Garcia-Villa J, Redondo-Ibanez M, Diaz Ramon C. Balloon Sphincteroplasty and Transpapillary Elimination of Bile Duct Stones: 10 Years' Experience. *AJR* 2004; 182: 1451-1458.

[35] Itoi T, Shinohara Y, Takeda K, et al., A novel technique for endoscopic sphincterotomy when using a percutaneous transhepatic cholangioscope in patients with an endoscopically inaccessible papilla. *Gastrointest. Endosc*. 2004; 59; 708–11.

[36] Ahmed A, Husain S, Saad N et al., Accessing the common bile duct after Roux-en-Y gastric bypass. *Surg. Obes. Relat. Dis*. 2007; 3: 640-3.

In: The Fundamentals of Bariatric Surgery
Editors: Shahzeer Karmali and Daniel W. Birch
ISBN: 978-1-62417-732-3

Chapter 16

Revisional Bariatric Surgery

Vadim Sherman and Michele Riordon
Methodist Hospital, Houston, TX, US

Abstract

Restrictive procedures have been a mainstay of bariatric surgery. Attaining an optimal level of restriction may result in significant weight loss success. However, failure of the restrictive operation due to weight regain or proximal gastric outlet obstruction may necessitiate conversion to another procedure. This chapter deals with the surgical options of revision surgery.

History

A number of restrictive procedures have been developed, each with varying success. They have in common the goal of reducing gastric capacity, inducing early satiety and maintaining intestinal continuity. One such procedure was conceived in the late 1970's by Wilkinson and Peloso. Using a 2 cm strip of marlex mesh, they created a non-adjustable gastric band around the upper part of the stomach. [1] After its initial introduction, variatrions were made by altering the implant material. These included the use of Dacron, silastic tubing and Gore-Tex mesh, amongst others. [2] Although a limited amount of patients found significant success with weight loss, the non-adjustable gastric band failed due to a number of complications. These included an inadequate stomal opening, erosion of the band, stomach prolapse, and multiple adverse gastrointestinal symptoms such as reflux, regurgitation, food intolerance, and intractable vomiting.

Over the same time period, another restrictive procedure, the vertical banded gastroplasty, came into existence. Developed by Mason, the operation involved the creation of a small pouch based off the lesser curvature. A window was created through the anterior and posterior walls of the stomach, near the incisura angularis. Through this window, a stapler was then applied in the direction of the angle of His. The stomach was stapled but not divided, resulting in the creation of a 50cc tubularized gastric pouch.

Table 1. late complications of LAGB requiring operative re-intervention

Complication	Frequency (%)
Band slippage	5.5 – 10.5
Band erosion	6.2 – 9.0
Severe esophageal dilatation	3.1 - 3.5
Severe food intolerance/reflux esophagitis	6.0 - 6.9
Leak (port/catheter/band)	8.4 – 10.0
Insufficient weight loss (<25% EWL at 5 years)	10.5 – 33.3

In addition, the outlet to the pouch was banded with a polypropylene collar to maintain a constant stomal diameter. [3] Another variation of this technique involves the use of a silastic ring to conform the outlet diameter. Instead of using a circular stapler to create an opening on the stomach, a prolene suture is placed through the lower end of the staple line and then around the lesser curvature. A pre-cut length of silastic tubing is then threaded over the stitch. A 32F Ewald tube stents the outlet as the stitch is tied [4]. As the procedure became widely accepted, a number of modifications ensued to maximize the extent of weight loss. This included narrowing the stomal diameter with shorter pieces of marlex mesh and silastic rings, as well as reducing the internal diameter of the pouch by stapling over smaller intragastric tubes. Overall, VBG resulted in significantly high long term complication rates (>35%) due to outlet obstruction, erosion of the band, staple line disruption, food intolerance, maladaptive eating, and weight regain. [5] The procedure ultimately fell out of favor.

The experience with non-adjustable gastric banding and vertical banded gastroplasty demonstrated that complications were usually due to gastric outlet obstruction at the band site. Whether the outlet was created intentionally too small or subsequent inflammatory response led to a stricturing at the band site, the problem with these restrictive operations was a lack of adjustability. To this end, a number of surgeons began developing an adjustable gastric band. Kuzmak first implanted his adjustable band in 1983 and it consisted of a silicone band reinforced by Dacron. The band volume could be adjusted through its connection to a subcutaneous port [6] Separately, Hallberg patented his ‘balloon band’ in Sweden in 1985. This became known as the Swedish Adjustable Gastric Band (SAGB). The early experience with the SAGB was to place the band through a laparotomy, however, in 1992, Forsell developed the laparoscopic adjustable gastric band placement. [7]

General Considerations

A failed restrictive bariatric procedure will generally present as a proximal gastric outlet obstruction and/or weight regain. Depending on the primary complaint, the patient may present with varying degrees of weight loss. The first step is to assess the patient’s gastrointestinal quality of life. This includes a detailed questionnaire focusing on specific food tolerances, dysphagia, and extent of other adverse symptoms such as vomiting, regurgitation and gastroesophageal reflux. The information gleaned from this survey will help understand the patient's eating habits. Inappropriate nutritional choices may be a consequence of a proximal gastric outlet obstruction at the band site. Patients will often present complaining of a paradox: "I can't eat anything, but I'm gaining weight". This common complaint illustrates well the concept of maladaptive eating. [8-10] In this situation, patients are unable to tolerate solid foods such as vegetables, breads and meats, thereby leading them to adopt a diet consisting of liquids and soft foods, which usually are calorie dense. Alternatively, patients with a significant degree of proximal gastric outlet obstruction may present with excessive weight loss secondary to inadequate nutrtional intake. Lastly, a patient may present with weight regain and no symptoms of proximal gastric outlet obstruction.

With respect to adjustable gastric banding specifically, experience over time has demonstrated a substantial long-term complication and failure rate requiring either revision of the gastric band or conversion to another procedure, despite the low incidence of perioperative complications[11-13].

The overall failure rate of the LAGB is up to 50% at 10 years. Almost one third of patients fail due inadequate weight loss defined as EWL of less than 25% and 40-50% have an EWL of less than 50% at long-term follow up. An additional 20 to 33% of patients have their band removed or are converted to another bariatric procedure at 10 year follow up due to gastric banding complications or inadequate weight loss. The LAGB late complications that require re-intervention and their rates of occurrence are summarized in Table 1. [14-18].

Diagnostic testing is essential when evaluation a patient for a possible revision and involves the use of both an EGD and UGI. An UGI is useful to document presence of reflux, hiatal hernia, esophageal dilatation, pouch dilatation, degree of stomal stenosis, and presence of vertical staple line breakdown (unique to VBG). [Figure 1, 2 and 3] An UGI is particularly useful to evaluate the adjustable gastric band position and possibility of slip. An EGD will complement the UGI with a better assessment of stomal stenosis, ability to measure the length of the pouch, and visualize a band erosion. [19, 20]. [Figure 4] Should a band erosion be identified, therapeutic endoscopic techniques can be used to remove the band. [21, 22] A dilatation at the band site is not useful as the band material is non-pliable and resists any stretching. Staple line disruption in VBG may result on its own or secondary to increased intra-pouch pressure from proximal gastric outlet obstruction. [23, 24].

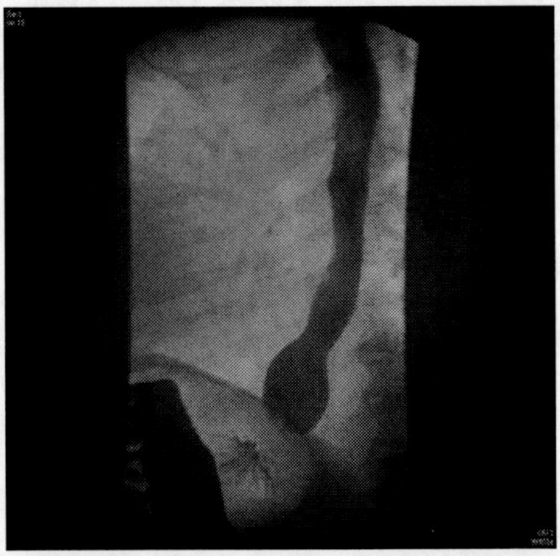

Figure 1. UGI of a patient with proximal gastric outlet obstruction following a nonadjustable gastric band.

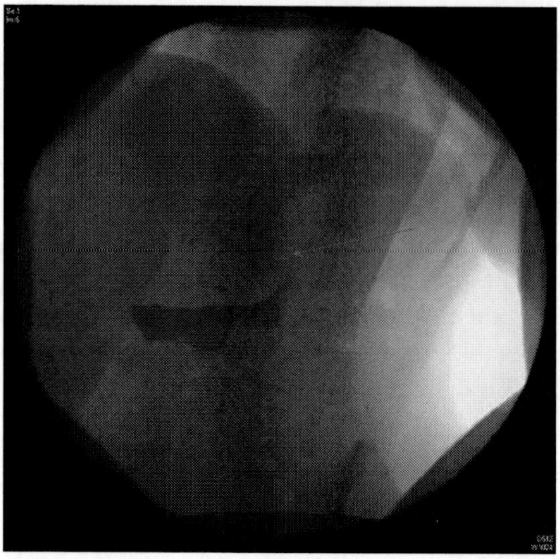

Figure 2. UGI of a patient with proximal gastric outlet obstruction at the silastic band of a VBG. Contrast fills the proximal pouch and slowly transits through the stoma into the antrum of the stomach.

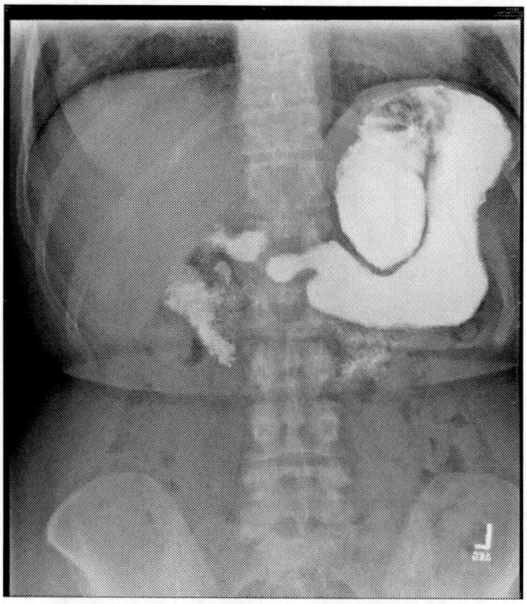

Figure 3. UGI demonstrating a gastro-gastric fistula secondary to staple line breakdown in a VBG.

A large staple line disruption provides a path of least resistance for ingested food, thereby obviating any restrictive effect of the vertical banded gastroplasty. Esophageal manometry may provide additional information about esophageal dysfunction, such as pseudoachalasia, although this is an uncommon consequence. [25]

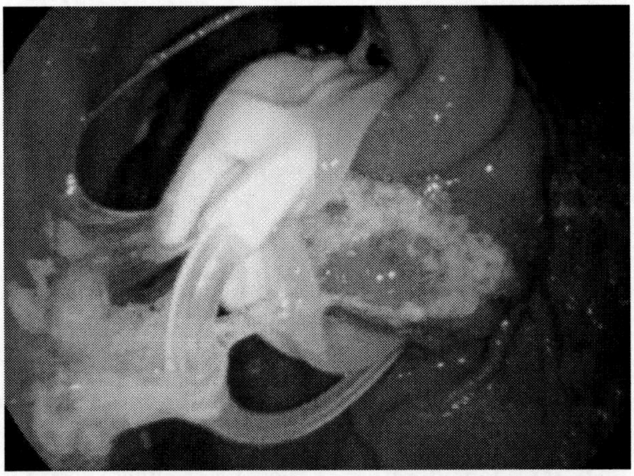

Figure 4. An eroded adjustable gastric band as seen on retroflexion during an EGD.

Operative Considerations

The authors advocate a conversion of VBG or NAGB to a Roux-en-Y gastric bypass. Reversal of the initial operation by band removal is another option to relieve symptoms of proximal gastric outlet obstruction, however, simple reversal will often result in weight regain. In regards to conversion of failed LAGB, choices of revision include sleeve gastrectomy or Roux-en-Y gastric bypass. Although the vertical banded gastroplasty operation was adapted to a laparoscopic operation, the majority of the procedures were performed using a midline laparotomy of variable length. Non-adjustable gastric bands were all placed using an open technique, whereas the overwhelming majority of adjustable gastric bands are placed laparoscoically. Subsequently, the surgeon must contend with significant, and often dense, intra-abdominal adhesions following VBG and NAGB. Nevertheless, the revision of a non-adjustable gastric band or vertical banded gastroplasty can be performed using laparoscopy. [26, 27]

VBG

Adhesions around the upper stomach are variable post VBG, yet they surely will involve an element of scar tissue between the left lobe of the liver and the site of the band. Once the omental adhesions have been cleared, sharp dissection is initiated to separate the liver from the stomach. Oftentimes, the liver capsule is entered and bleeding is encountered.

With the left lobe of the liver retracted, the stomach anatomy can be examined and the components of the vertical banded gastroplasty can be identified. The site of the band can be identified by the abundance of scar tissue around it, especially if the band consists of marlex mesh. Should the band be made from silastic tubing, palpation with an instrument will help identify it and its surrounding capsule.

Once the location of the band is clear, the vertical staple line can be identified as progressing from the band site to the angle of His. If the staple line was plicated with a modified fundoplication, the short gastric vessels may be found along the anterior aspect of the stomach. Careful dissection with an advanced energy source must be performed in order to avoid blood loss from the short gastrics. Sharp dissection is then performed in order to return the greater curve to its normal anatomical position, thereby exposing the vertical staple line.

Adhesions along the lesser curvature will complicate the entry into the lesser sac. Therefore, entry into the lesser sac is gained via the greater curvature. Once the left gastric artery is identified, a window along the lesser curvature can be created. The authors advocate a partial gastrectomy as part of the conversion procedure. This involves removal of the portion of the stomach containing the band and the vertical staple line. The pouch is created by stapling proximal to the level of the gastric band and medial to the vertical staple line. The portion of stomach between the new staple line and the old vertical staple line may not drain effectively, especially in the setting of stomal stenosis. Resection of this segment thereby removes this concern. Another consideration is that the stomach tissue is likely to be scarred and the appropriate stapler cartridge should be chosen to accommodate the thickened tissue. Lastly, the pouch can be formed over a bougie or endoscope to ensure adequate sizing. A gastrostomy tube in the excluded stomach is not routinely advocated.

Another consideration is the presence of a hiatal hernia. With a long standing obstruction, the pouch may dilate and a hiatal hernia may also result. Preoperative studies will identify whether this is the case. If a hiatal hernia is encountered intra-operatively, a crural repair should be performed concurrently with the conversion. The crural repair should be performed in a standard fashion, with circumferential dissection around the distal esophagus, mobilization of the GEJ into the abdominal space, and closure of the crural defect with permanent suture.

Foillowing the creation of the gastric pouch, the jejuno-jejunostomy is performed in a standard fashion. The gastro-jejunal anastomosis is then performed. The authors advocate using a linear stapling or completely hand sewn technique. Use of a circular stapler may be difficult if the tissue is thickened.

Non-adjustable Gastric Band

Non-adjustable gastric bands were generally placed through small upper midline incisions. Despite the deceivingly small skin incision, patients may have a variable amount of omental adhesions. The adhesions of the liver to the capsule around the band, however, will likely be very dense, secondary to the desmoplastic reaction with the band material, often Dacron or Marlex. Access to the stomach and band must first be preceded by lysing adhesions between the upper stomach and liver. Once the left lobe of the liver is retracted, the band can be identified. An intra-operative endoscopy may be useful to confirm the band location in situations where the inflammatory tissue is dense enough to prevent laparoscopic palpation. Once the band is identified, the lesser curve is dissected such that a window into the lesser sac is gained above and below the level of the band.

The size of the proximal pouch may be variable, depending on the initial location of placement of the band and the subsequent pouch dilatation resulting from obstruction at the band site. Regardless, the stomach should be transected proximal to the band site in order to avoid incorporating the strictured and thickened portion of the stomach. Prior to transecting the stomach, the band capsule can be entered and the band carefully removed from around the stomach. The dense inflammatory tissue may make band removal difficult without performing an inadvertent enterotomy. In those sitatuions, the option is to remove the anterior portion of the band, remove as much secondary scar tissue and then transect the stomach just proximal to the band. Otherwise, the portion of the stomach including the band can be resected. This is especially indicated if the degree of obstruction at the band site will prevent adequate drainage of the cut end of the stomach into the remainder of the excluded stomach. Once the pouch has been created, the remainder of the Roux-en-Y gastric bypass is performed. Unlike the conversion of a VBG, the proximal gastric pouch is shortened and the stomach tissue is much thicker around the site of the band. Special considerations must therefore be taken when transecting the upper stomach with a stapler, as the tissue thickness may be prohibitive to routine transection. Similar to VBG conversion, the authors advocate a linear stapler or hand sewn technique when creating the gastro-jejunostomy.

Adjustable Gastric Band

Adhesions secondary to adjustable gastric banding are usually minimal. The band tubing is easily identified within the abdomen and subsequently traced to the buckle of the band. Electrocautery is useful to open the capsule directly over the buckle of the band, thereby obviating any injury to surrounding structures. Once the capsule is opened, the gastropexy can be identified and carefully dissected using sharp dissection. The gastropexy sutures are a good guide to identify the plane between the fundus and the proximal stomach. The gastropexy should be completely dissected such that the stomach can be returned to its near normal anatomical position.

The gastric band is then transected using endoscopic scissors and the band is gently removed from its location. The gastric pouch is then formed. If the proximal stomach has minimal scar tissue, a gastric pouch can be formed based off the left gastric artery. If there is a significant stricture at the level of the band, the endoscopic stapler can be placed at or slightly above the level of the band, in order to create a pouch proximal to the level of the obstruction. A special consideration is made when dividing the stomach near the angle of His- the tissue is thickest here, secondary to scar tissue and appropriate changes must be made in stapler cartridge. The gastric band is placed aside for retrieval at the end of the case. The Roux-en-Y gastric bypass is then performed in the standard fashion.

If the adjustable gastric band is revised to a sleeve gastrectomy, particular attention must be paid at the proximal stomach. Transection of the proximal stomach is technically more difficult than a primary sleeve gastrectomy secondary to the thickened and scarred gastric tissue. This will necessitate an appropriately thick stapler cartridge. Stapling laterall to the angle of His to avoid this thickened tissue is not normally advised as it is likely to result in a retained fundal pouch, proximal to the remainder of the tubularized stomach. This retained portion may subsequently lead to inadequate restriction and the possibility of retained food and gastric secretions.

Outcomes

VBG Conversion to RYGB

Various studies have cited that between 35-55% of VBG patients have ultimately undergone revision surgery. [28, 29] With regards to resolution of symptoms of proximal gastric outlet obstruction, conversion of VBG to RYGB has been shown to be effective in resolving GERD. In a series of 28 VBG patients with GERD, conversion to RYGB was associated with a resolution of symptoms in 86%. [19] Several studies have examined the effect of revision of the VBG versus conversion to RYGB for weight regain. The largest study of VBG revisions involved 101 patients, 74 of which underwent conversion to Roux-en-Y gastric bypass. Patients undergoing conversion to RYGB did have a significant weight loss, with a BMI drop from 40.5 kg/m2 to 30.1 kg/m2.. However, the revisions were associated with a high complication rate (55%). [30] As the volume of revisional surgery continues to grow and the familiarity with the procedure increases, the complication rate will likely improve. In a study by Gagner et al, the complication rate was shown to be 8%. [31] Nevertheless, the surgeon performing conversions of VBG to RYGB must be prepared to deal with anastomotic leak, bleeding, stricturing, and marginal ulceration at a higher rate compared to primary RYGB surgery.

AGB Conversion to RYGB

The most common reason for conversion of AGB to RYGB is inadequate loss or weight regain. [32, 33] Several studies have shown conversion of AGB to RYGB to be safe and efficacious. The average percentage of EWL at time of conversion is 23%. At 12 months after conversion, patients achieve EWL ranging between 50% and 57% based on their pre-AGB weight. [34-36] A retrospective review of 75 patients since then by Lim confirms the weight loss benefit after conversion. [37]A study by Gagne combined results of revision to RYGB after failed ABG from the 4 largest series published at that time and found an overall complication rate of 7% (range 0-19%). Complications include wound infection, intestinal hemorrhage, fever, small bowel obstruction requiring surgery, staple line leaks, intra-abdominal abscesses and pneumonia. [33]

AGB Conversion to SG

Conversion of an adjustable gastric band to another restrictive procedure such sleeve gastrectomy occurs less frequently than conversion to RYGB. It is a reasonable revision choice if there are no contraindications such as gastric dysmotility, esophageal dysfunction or reflux esophagitis. There are no long term results available, however Foletto et al, published a series of 52 patients who underwent revision of AGB to SG primarily for inadequate weight loss. At 2 years follow-up, the mean EWL was 41.6%. This seems to indicate that it is effective as a revisional procedure but the complication rate was much higher when compared to conversion to RYGB. There was a 1.9% mortality rate, 5.7% perigastric hematoma rate, and 5.7% leak rate. [38]

Conclusion

Restrictive bariatric procedures may fail due to weight regain and/or proximal gastric outlet obstruction. Patients that are possible candidates for a revision of their previous bariatric procedure must be investigated with an UGI and EGD to assess their anatomy and define the degree of proximal gastric outlet obstruction. Furthermore, old operative reports should be obtained, along with a diet and GI quality of life questionnaire, in order to fully understand the patient's reason for failure. Once the decision to proceed with the revision has been made, the operation of choice is a conversion to a Roux-en-Y gastric bypass. Other surgical options include reversal of the restrictive procedure.

References

[1] Wilkinson, L.H. and O.A. Peloso, Gastric (reservoir) reduction for morbid obesity. *Arch. Surg.*, 1981. 116(5): p. 602-5.

[2] Oria, H.E., Gastric segmentation: nonadjustable banding by minilaparotomy: historical review. *Surg. Obes. Relat. Dis.*, 2009. 5(3): p. 365-70.

[3] Mason, E.E., Vertical banded gastroplasty for obesity. *Arch. Surg.*, 1982. 117(5): p. 701-6.

[4] Laws, H.L. and S. Piantadosi, Superior gastric reduction procedure for morbid obesity: a prospective, randomized trial. *Ann. Surg.*, 1981. 193(3): p. 334-40.

[5] Mason, E.E., Development and future of gastroplasties for morbid obesity. *Arch. Surg.*, 2003. 138(4): p. 361-6.

[6] Kuzmak, L.I., A Review of Seven Years' Experience with Silicone Gastric Banding. *Obes. Surg.*, 1991. 1(4): p. 403-408.

[7] McBride, C.L. and V. Kothari, Evolution of laparoscopic adjustable gastric banding. *Surg. Clin. North Am.* 91(6): p. 1239-47, viii-ix.

[8] Kriwanek, S., et al., Dietary changes after vertical banded gastroplasty. *Obes. Surg.*, 2000. 10(1): p. 37-40.

[9] Ikramuddin, S., T.A. Kellogg, and D.B. Leslie, Laparoscopic conversion of vertical banded gastroplasty to a Roux-en-Y gastric bypass. *Surg. Endosc.*, 2007. 21(11): p. 1927-30.

[10] del Amo, D.A., et al., Vertical banded gastroplasty: is it a durable operation for morbid obesity? *Obes. Surg.*, 2004. 14(4): p. 536-8.

[11] Fielding, G.A., Rhodes, M., Nathanson, L.K., Laparoscopic gastric banding for morbid obesity: surgical outcome in 335 cases. *Surg. Endosc.*, 1999. 13: p. 550-54.

[12] Suter, M., Bettschart, V., Giusti, V., Heraief, E., Jayet, A., A 3-year experience with laparoscopic gastric banding for obesity. *Surg. Endosc.*, 2000. 14: p. 532-36.

[13] Dargent, J., Laparoscopic adjustable gastric banding: lessons from the first 500 patients in a single institution. *Obes. Surg.* 1999. 9(5): p. 446-52.

[14] Martikainen, T., et al., Long-term results, complications and quality of life in a seriers of adjustable gastric banding. *Obes. Surg*. 2004. 14: p. 648-54.
[15] Spivak, H., Abdelmelek, M.F., Beltran, O.R., Ng, A.W., Kitahama, S., Long-term outcomes of laparoscopic adjustable gastric banding and laparoscopic roux-en-y gastric bypass in the United States. *Surg. Endosc*. 2012.
[16] Suter, M., Calmes, J.M., Paroz, A., Giusti, V., A 10-year experience with laparoscopic gastric banding for morbid obesity: high long-term complication and failure rates. *Obes. Surg*. 2006. 16: p. 829-35.
[17] Bueter, M., et al., Short and long-term results of laparoscopic gastric banding for morbid obesity. *Langenbecks Arch. Surg*. 2008. 393: p. 199-205.
[18] Zuegel, N.P., et al., Complications and outcome after laparoscopic bariatric surgery: LAGB versus LRYGB. *Langenbecks Arch. Surg*. 2012.
[19] Gonzalez, R., et al., Operative technique for converting a failed vertical banded gastroplasty to Roux-en-Y gastric bypass. *J. Am. Coll. Surg*., 2005. 201(3): p. 366-74.
[20] Behrns, K.E., et al., Reoperative bariatric surgery. Lessons learned to improve patient selection and results. *Ann. Surg*., 1993. 218(5): p. 646-53.
[21] Karmali, S., et al., Endoscopic management of eroded prosthesis in vertical banded gastroplasty patients. *Surg. Endosc*. 24(1): p. 98-102.
[22] Karmali, S., et al., Transgastric endoscopic rendezvous technique for removal of eroded Molina gastric band. *Surg. Obes. Relat. Dis*., 2008. 4(4): p. 559-62.
[23] Melissas, J., et al., Staple-line disruption following vertical banded gastroplasty. *Obes. Surg*., 1998. 8(1): p. 15-20.
[24] Svenheden, K.E., et al., Staple disruption in vertical banded gastroplasty. *Obes. Surg*., 1997. 7(2): p. 136-8; discussion 139-41.
[25] Seymour, K., et al., Changes in esophageal function after vertical banded gastroplasty as demonstrated by esophageal scintigraphy. *Obes. Surg*., 1998. 8(4): p. 429-33.
[26] Iannelli, A., et al., Laparoscopic conversion of vertical banded gastroplasty with an antireflux wrap into Roux-en-Y gastric bypass. *Obes. Surg*., 2007. 17(7): p. 901-4.
[27] Gagne, D.J., E. Dovec, and J.E. Urbandt, Laparoscopic revision of vertical banded gastroplasty to Roux-en-Y gastric bypass: outcomes of 105 patients. *Surg. Obes. Relat. Dis*. 7(4): p. 493-9.
[28] Cohen, R., et al., Laparoscopic revisional bariatric surgery: myths and facts. *Surg. Endosc*., 2005. 19(6): p. 822-5.
[29] Benotti, P.N. and R.A. Forse, Safety and long-term efficacy of revisional surgery in severe obesity. *Am. J. Surg*., 1996. 172(3): p. 232-5.
[30] Schouten, R., et al., Conversion of vertical banded gastroplasty to Roux-en-Y gastric bypass results in restoration of the positive effect on weight loss and co-morbidities: evaluation of 101 patients. *Obes. Surg*., 2007. 17(5): p. 622-30.
[31] Gagner, M., et al., Laparoscopic reoperative bariatric surgery: experience from 27 consecutive patients. *Obes. Surg*., 2002. 12(2): p. 254-60.
[32] Ardestani, A., Lautz, D.B., Tavakkolizadeh, A., Band revision versis roux-en-y gastric bypass conversion as salvage operation after laparoscopic adjustable gastric banding. *Surg. Obes. Relat. Dis*. 2011. 7(1): p. 33-7.
[33] Gagner, M., Gumbs, A.A., Gastric banding: conversion to sleeve, bypass, or DS. *Surg. Endosc*. 2007. 21:p 1931-5.

[34] Moore, R., Perugini, R., Czerniach, D., Gallagher-Dorval, K., Mason, R., Kelly, J.J., Early results of conversion of laparoscopic adjustable gastric band to roux-en-y gastric bypass. *Surg. Obes. Relat. Dis.* 2009. 5(4):p. 439-43.

[35] Weber, M., et al., Laparoscopic roux-en-y gastric bypass, but not rebanding, should be proposed as rescue procedure for patients with failed laparoscopic gastric banding. *Ann. Surg*. 2003. 328(6):p. 827-33.

[36] Langer, F.B., et al., Inadequate weight loss vs secondary weight regain: laparoscopic conversion from gastric banding to roux-en-y gastric bypass. *Obes. Surg.* 2008. 18(11):p. 1381-6.

[37] Lim, C. S. H., Liew, V., Talbot, M.L., Jorgensen, J. O., Loi, K. W., Revisional bariatric surgery. *Obes. Surg*. 2009. 19:p. 827-32.

[38] Foletto, M., et al., Sleeve gastrectomy as revisional procedure for failed gastric banding or gastroplasty. *Surg. Obes. Relat. Dis*. 2010. 6(2): p. 146-51.

In: The Fundamentals of Bariatric Surgery
Editors: Shahzeer Karmali and Daniel W. Birch
ISBN: 978-1-62417-732-3

Chapter 17

Body Contouring after Massive Weight Loss

Warren A. Ellsworth and Jeffrey D. Friedman
The Institute for Reconstructive Surgery, Methodist Hospital, Houston, TX, US
Division of Plastic Surgery, Weill Cornell Medical College, New York, NY, US
Division of Plastic Surgery, Baylor College of Medicine, Houston, TX, US
Division of Plastic Surgery, Methodist Hospital, Houston, TX, US

Abstract

The number of patients interested in body contouring surgery after massive weight loss continues to grow. The diversity of body types has created an entire sub-specialty of plastic surgical procedures dedicated to improving form and function in these patients. Appropriate pre-operative work up is essential to the success of surgical treatment due to common nutritional deficiencies and medical co-morbidities. Of equal importance is a lengthy discussion of the scars required to improve the patient's contour, the number of surgical procedures required to achieve the patient's goals, and the length of recovery involved with each stage of treatment.

In our center, total body contouring is performed in a staged fashion due to the lengthy operative and recovery times required for successful re-shaping of the skin and tissue. The central trunk is often addressed first, as this is the area of biggest concern for the majority of patients. In secondary and tertiary surgical procedures, the upper body, arms, breasts and medial thighs are treated. Each stage is personalized toward the degree of soft tissue deflation and aesthetic goals of the patient.

Common complications such as seroma development and wound dehiscence should be mitigated by the judicious use of drains and tensionless layered closure, respectively. Ultimately, patient satisfaction after body contouring surgery is quite high. Many patients find a new confidence as they discover that their outer appearance finally reflects their more youthful and healthy inner self, which they discovered after weight loss.

Introduction

As bariatric surgery for treatment of obesity has gained popularity, the number of patients seeking improvement in body contour after massive weight loss has grown significantly. These patients present at various points during their weight loss with significant deflation of the tissues of the face, trunk and extremities. Although each patient has a unique set of aesthetic challenges, the psychological complaint is always similar – the patient looks and feels thinner but still cannot enjoy their new body due to redundant skin that not only limits their confidence and their ability to wear certain clothes but may also present hygiene issues related to chronic intertrigo. Removal of excess skin and subcutaneous tissue through contouring procedures offers the massive weight loss patient a completion of their weight loss journey and in some instances reduce the medical risks associated with severely redundant skin.

Timing and Work Up

Patients present to the plastic surgeon for body contouring procedures at all stages of weight loss. Often patients who are still in the active weight loss stage will inquire about liposuction and abdominoplasty. Most plastic surgeons will agree, however, that surgical intervention should be delayed until the patient reaches his or her goal weight and has maintained that weight for at least 6 months time. For a host of reasons, many bariatric patients come close to but do not reach their ideal weight. For these cases, the surgeon must use judgment and evaluate the degree of tissue "deflation" and goals of the patient to determine the most appropriate timing for surgical intervention.

Although many patients enjoy significant improvement in their medical co-morbidities after bariatric surgery, all still deserve a complete work-up prior to elective and lengthy body contouring procedures. Nutritional deficiencies should be identified early and treated well before embarking on these cosmetic procedures as metabolic abnormalities are often seen many years after bariatric procedures. Any history of heart disease, diabetes and smoking is of special importance to the plastic surgeon and impacts the patient's ability to heal the large wounds associated with body contouring surgery. The mental health of the massive weight loss patient should be assessed as well. Many of these men and women have had significant emotional and psychiatric problems throughout their life, and a visit with a psychiatrist for evaluation and clearance is often warranted.

The initial exam of the massive weight loss patient should include a detailed evaluation of the degree of weight loss, skin laxity, deflation, and previous surgical scars. (Figures 1A, 1B) Pinching tissues in the arm, breast, abdomen and thighs can allow for the surgeon to estimate the degree of tissue laxity and amount of resection possible. After performing a thorough exam, it is essential to determine the patient's goals and priorities. While the patient will complain about his or her entire body, when pressed for the area that is most disturbing, he or she will often point to the abdomen and central trunk region.

In our opinion, body contouring surgery for the massive weight loss patient is safely performed in a staged fashion due to the lengthy operative and recovery time required for successful re-shaping of the skin and tissue. We generally start with the area that offends the patient most significantly and then outline a series of staged procedures that will achieve the goals of the patient in a safe and effective fashion. Often the central trunk will be treated in a first stage with a "body lift" or circumferential abdominoplasty procedure.

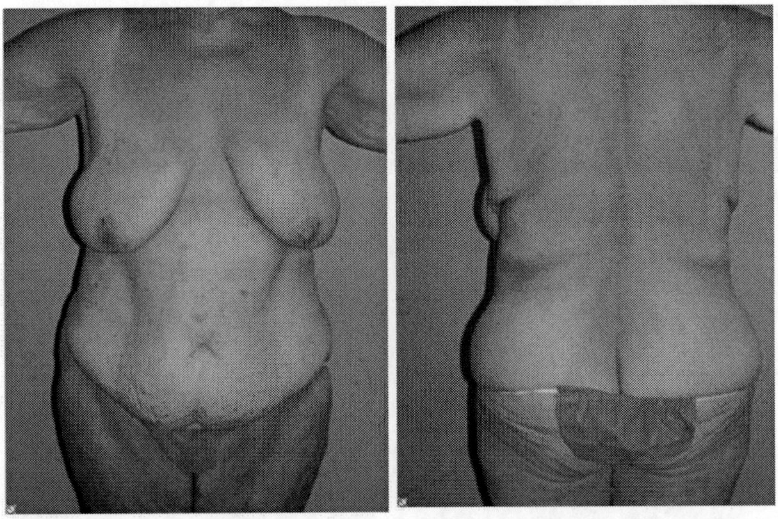

A B

Figures 1A, 1B. Patient after massive weight loss exhibiting soft tissue ptosis of the breasts, anterior and posterior trunk as well as thighs.

The second stage often treats the upper trunk/breasts and arms. Finally, the medial thighs and face can be addressed as needed and in accordance with the patient's wishes. With each stage, the patient must be well aware of the incisions planned and the drains required to successfully achieve their transformation. Recovery can take several weeks and wound healing difficulty and seroma formation is common and should be discussed prior to any surgical intervention.

The Lower Trunk

The appearance of the central abdomen in the massive weight loss patient varies greatly and usually includes both vertical and horizontal excess of skin and fat and ptosis of the pubic mound. (Figures 1A, 1B) In the aesthetic ideal, the contour of the trunk narrows just above the umbilicus at the level of the waist. While this occurs to a lesser degree in men, some narrowing is aesthetically pleasing. With this in mind, the goal of this stage of surgery is to remove the deflated skin and return the patient to a more normal shape. The trade off, of course is a large scar.

In the traditional massive weight loss patient who has successfully lost over 100 pounds, the degree of tissue deflation is best treated by a circumferential excision of skin and fat – this technique not only allows for removal of redundant tissue but also "lifting" of areas that have become ptotic during the deflation that occurs with weight loss. Areas that often benefit from this lifting technique include the lateral thighs as well as the buttocks.

We utilize a "pinch test" to see how far up the skin can move on the central abdomen, the lateral thighs as well as the buttocks – this allows for determination of the degree of soft tissue translation and the amount of tissue that can safely be removed. Patients who have not reached their ideal BMI and still retain a significant amount of subcutaneous fat will not tolerate as significant skin resection due to the thickness of the tissue. On the contrary, those patients who have achieved their goal weight and have significant "deflation" of their skin envelope will require significant removal of skin to achieve the desired contour – these are the ideal patients for the body lift procedure.

The circumferential body lift procedure is lengthy and can be associated with significant blood loss. For these reasons medical clearance preoperatively is generally a requirement. Once nutritionally and medically optimized the patient is planned for surgery. A lengthy discussion about the location of surgical incisions, drains required, length of recovery, and time off of work should be part of every pre-operative discussion. The most common complications remain formation of seroma and wound healing difficulty, which should be highlighted prior to surgery.

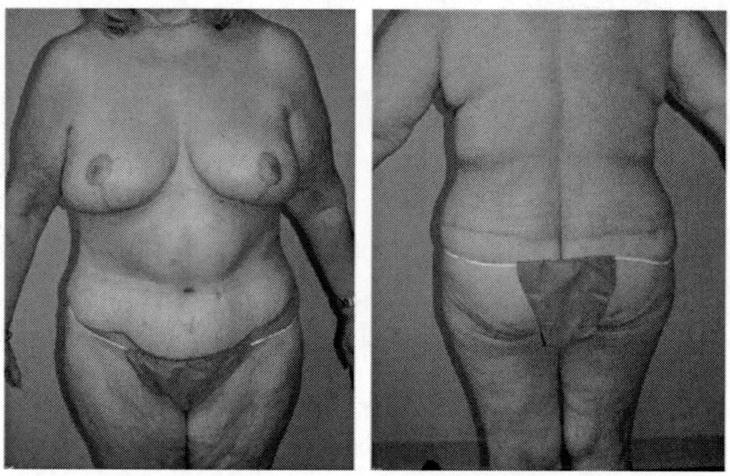

Figures 2A, 2B. Anterior and Posterior views after body lift procedure and mastopexy.

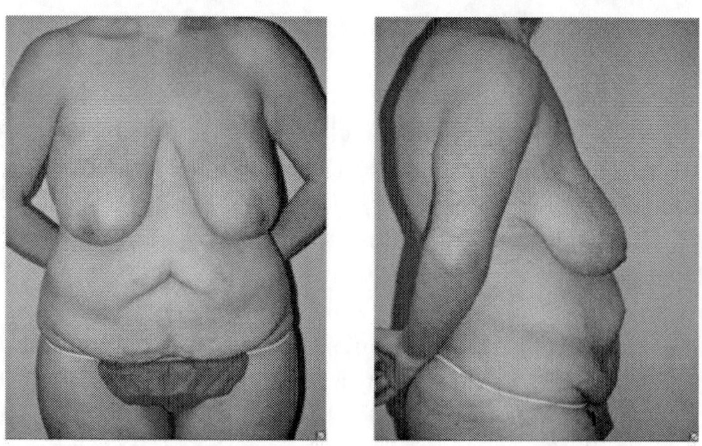

A B

Figures 3A, 3B. Patient after massive weight loss with significant decent of breast tissue as well as anterior trunk.

Perhaps the most important part of the surgical procedure occurs before the patient is put to sleep and prior to entering the operative theater. Accurate and thoughtful preoperative marking of the patient cannot be overemphasized. The marking is done with the patient in the standing position and outlines the area for resection and the location of the resultant scars. The three most important tenants to marking a patient for body lift procedure have been well outlined Aly [1] and are as follows: (1) The abdominoplasty part of the body lift should be maximized over resection of tissue on the back – this area is most visible to the patient; (2) The lateral resection should be maximized to achieve elevation of the lateral thighs; (3) The back resection, while important, should not be allowed to limit your resection on the abdomen. Therefore, the back is marked with the patient in the flexed position. Using these ideals, a marking pen is used to outline the area that is pinched for resection. Ideally the eventual scar is kept as low as possible to allow for hiding under swim wear and undergarments.

There are many different positional protocols for performing a body lift procedure. Some surgeons prefer starting supine and then prone while other prefer a lateral decubitus to lateral decubitus position. Regardless, at least one position change is required in a body lift, and at our center we prefer beginning prone and transitioning to supine to complete the body lift. After anterior skin resection, the fascia can be plicated centrally if needed to achieve a narrower waist line. Finally, the skin is closed in layers over several drains. Post operatively the patients are rapidly mobilized and expected to ambulate with assistance in the flexed position by post-operative day one. Prophylaxis against venous thrombo-embolic events is important in these patients, and we utilize sequential compression devices during and after surgery and use low molecular weight heparin daily for one week beginning on post-operative day one. Most patients are hospitalized for 1-2 days after surgery and most are able to stand straight up after 1-2 weeks. Follow up requires weekly evaluation of the drains and incisions, and the patients are usually released back to work and full activity by 4-6 weeks. (Figures 2A, 2B)

Upper Body and Breasts

Skin redundancy in the upper torso can occur either in isolation or in conjunction with lower trunk excess in the massive weight loss patient. If needed, upper body skin laxity is often treated in a second stage and follows the same principles as lower trunk surgery. Excess skin of the upper torso is resected and surgical scars are hidden within normal anatomic landmarks such as the inframammary fold.

In the female patient who has lost a significant amount of weight, breast ptosis and deflation is often a significant problem. (Figures 3A, 3B) Women complain that their breasts hang too low and that the upper pole is flat. To address these two major problems (volume loss and skin excess) we often perform mastopexy (breast lift) in conjunction with augmentation, to replace the tissue that has wasted away with weight loss. Some surgeons have described autologous methods of increasing breast volume, utilizing excess skin and fat of the lateral chest. More commonly, however, an implant is required to give a more youthful appearance to the breast. Further, in the massive weight loss patient plastic surgeons often delay the augmentation until a second stage in order to avoid devascularization of the breast and the catastrophic complication of nipple necrosis. In those patients who have sufficient residual breast volume, a mastopexy may be all that is required. (Figures 4A, 4B) As with any body contouring procedure, these women must understand the associated incisions required and scars that can be expected after this procedure. While it varies greatly due to the diversity of problems seen, most massive weight loss patients will require Wise pattern skin reduction, which results in scars around that areola, vertically down to the chest and along the inframammary fold. Woman, usually, are quite happy to trade these scars for a significant improvement in breast shape.

In men, breast excess is treated with several different methods depending on the degree of skin and soft tissue excess. This ranges from mild cases that require making incisions around the areola to more severe cases, which require amputation of breast tissue with free nipple grafting. It is, however increasingly hard to hide these often large and unsightly scars on the middle of the male chest. Unlike the female counterpart, there is no ptotic breast to hide the large transverse incisions. This requires significant discussion prior to any surgical procedure. However, in these cases of severe breast ptosis, the tradeoff is a small price to pay in order to achieve a more aesthetic appearance.

Upper and Lower Extremities

Excess skin of the proximal arm is a common area of concern from the weight loss patient. (Figures 5A, 5B) Procedures to address the upper extremity is often combined with upper body lift and/or breast surgery due to ease of access and proximity. The majority of massive weight loss patients require a full brachioplasty, or longitudinal excision of skin and fat with the scar canceled either under the arm or posteriorly. There remains considerable debate regarding the ideal position of the longitudinal scar. Many surgeons favor a scar along the medial aspect of the arm while others like the scar positioned along the posterior arm. (Figure 6A, 6B) Rarely, a massive weight loss patient will have minimal skin laxity and only require a "mini-brachioplasty," which is a procedure that can successfully remove a mild to moderate amount of skin redundancy while using only a small scar in the axilla. (Figures 7A, 7B)

As with all body contouring operations, the procedure begins with the patient awake and in the seated or standing position. Pre operative markings of the arms outline the extent of tissue resection and are estimated by pinching the excess tissue of the arm with the patients shoulders abducted to 90 degrees and elbows fully extended. After marking this first ellipse of tissue, one must account for the extra circumference needed to successfully close the wound after resection. To adjust for this, a second ellipse is drawn within the original resection outline. This area is usually 1-2 centimeters smaller in diameter and when resected will allow for translation and closure. [2] Usually patients are pleased with the improved contour and their new found ability to fit into shirts and dresses. Long scars are required and this should be discussed at length with the patient pre-operatively. Further if the skin and fat resection extends onto the chest wall, a "Z-Plasty" in the axilla is required to avoid scar contracture and limitations of range of motion at the shoulder joint post-operatively.

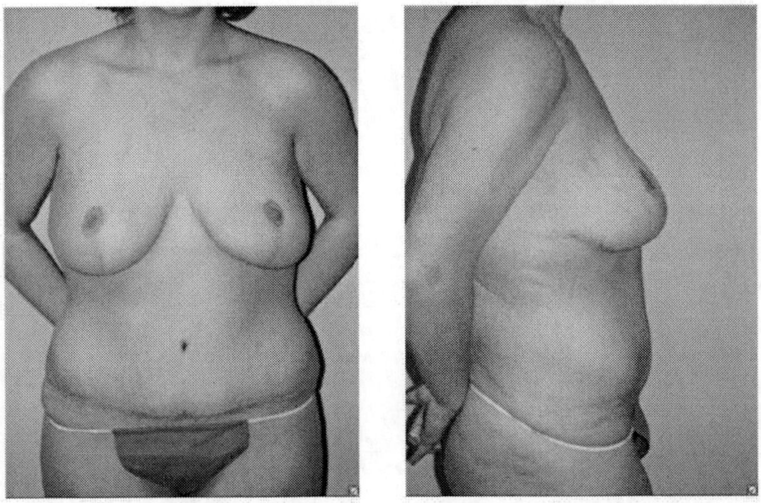

A B

Figures 4A, 4B. Anterior and Lateral view after mastopexy for repositioning and reshaping of the breast, as well as abdominoplasty for contouring of the anterior trunk.

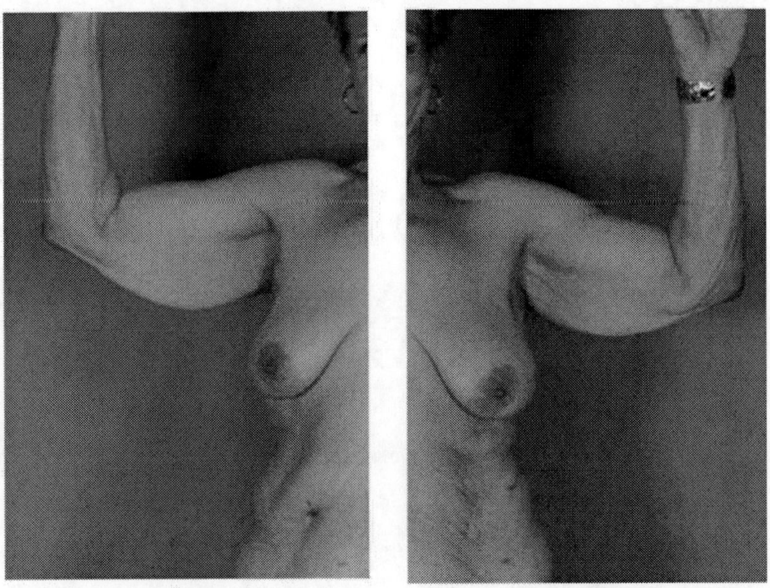

A B

Figures 5A, 5B. Massive weight loss patient exhibiting severe laxity of the entire arm from elbow to axilla.

The lateral portion of the lower extremity is often significantly improved during the initial "body-lift" stage as discussed early in this chapter. The medial thigh, however, is an area of great concern to many massive weight loss patients and often requires surgical intervention if improvement is desired. As with the upper extremity, the degree of laxity will determine the extent of surgery. If a small degree of skin laxity is apparent, a crecenteric excision parallel to the perineal crease can be sufficient.

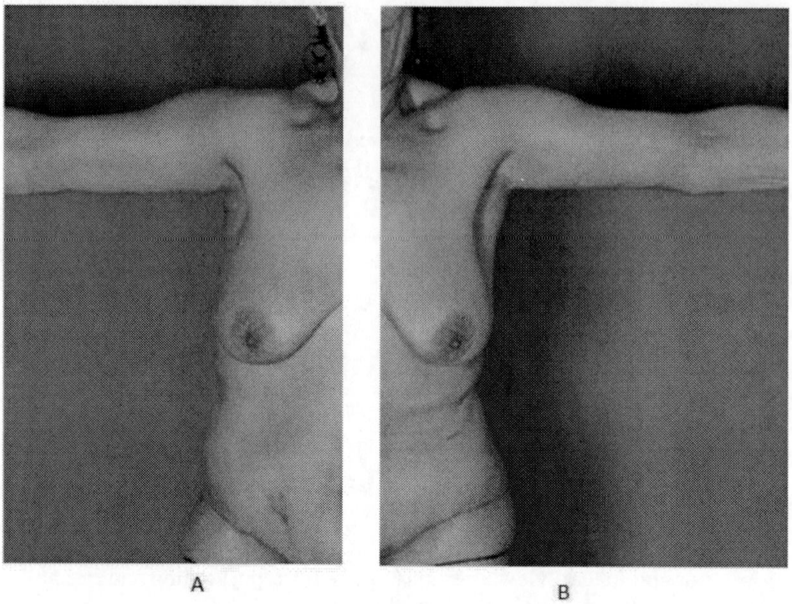

Figures 6A, 6B. Post operative photo after longitudinal resection of skin and fat with scar hidden in the posterior aspect of the arm.

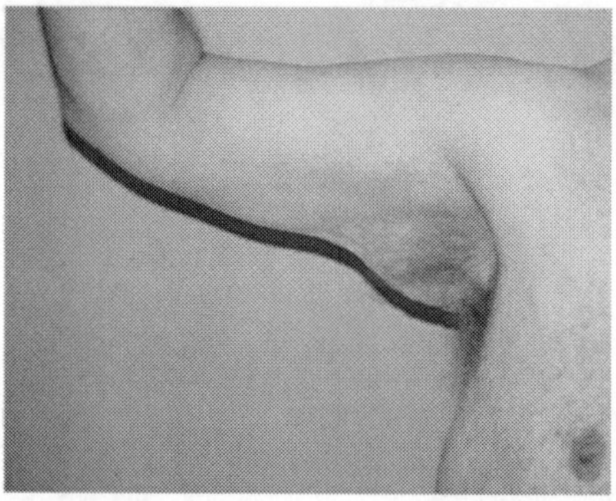

Figure 7A. Pre operative photo of massive weight loss patient with minimal laxity of the proximal arm.

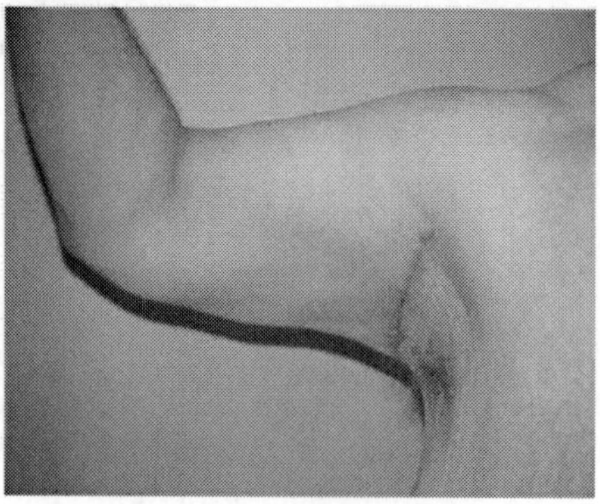

Figure 7B. Post operative photo after "mini" brachioplasty with incision in the axilla.

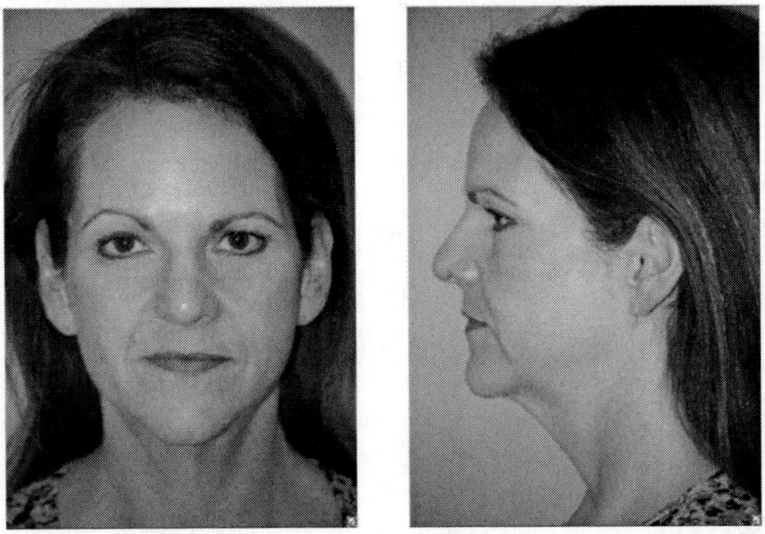

A B

Figures 8A, 8B. Patient after massive weight loss demonstrating decent and ptosis of the neck.

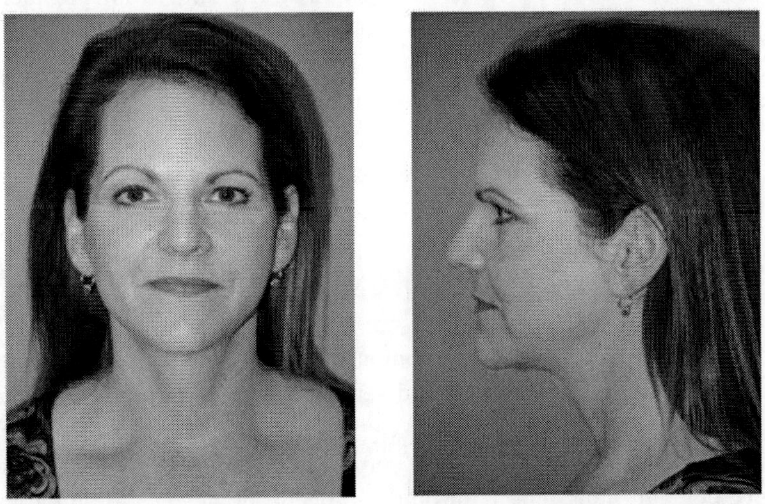

A B

Figures 9A, 9B. Post operative views of improved contour of jaw line after neck lift procedure.

The complication of labial spreading can occur if significant skin is resected in this vector. To avoid this complication, a longitudinal elliptical excision can be planned, tightening the cone of the lower extremity. Additionally, securing the flap at the femoral junction to the underlying fascia is central to avoiding decent of the scar and helps to avoid tension on the labia. In an identical fashion to the arm, an area of redundancy is pinched and marked in the medial thigh along the longitudinal plane. An ellipse is outlined based on the degree of skin redundancy. Again a smaller ellipse is planned within the larger outlined area to allow for less tension at closure. Resection is completed in the suprafascial plane, and special attention must be given as one approaches the proximal thigh as lymph nodes in this area are easily damaged. To avoid injury to this drainage plexus, transition to a more superficial dissection is required.

Closure in the medial thigh is similar to the arm. Layered closure over drains will help prevent seroma collection. The complication of lymphocele is dramatically reduced with special attention to the dissection in the proximal leg. Poor scaring is of course a possible complication, and this particular location is outside the normal area where undergarments cover. As such, a frank discussion about locations and length of scars is important.

Face and Neck

Usually the last area surgically treated in the massive weight loss patient is the face and neck. Just as in other anatomic areas, the face and neck can become deflated and ptotic with weight loss. (Figures 8A, 8B) Excess skin in this region prematurely ages a patient and can give a tired and lethargic appearance. Treatment often requires a full facelift, with incisions in front of the ear, behind the ear and along the posterior hairline. Occasionally, a small incision under the chin will allow for reconstruction of the platysma and removal of fat as well. After undermining the skin of the face and neck, the superficial musculo-appanurotic system (SMAS) is treated. This anatomic layer that separates the skin from the facial nerve and musculature is often plicated or lifted, thus repositioned to reshape the face in a youthful fashion. Ultimately, the skin is re-draped and excess removed. (Figures 9A, 9B) Special considerations must be given in this area to achieve a tensionless closure. If any significant tension is apparent at the time of skin closure, widened scars will occur and can brand the patient's face with many of the obvious signs of having had facelift surgery.

Complications

The overall complication rate of body contouring procedures can be quite high. Common complications include wound dehiscence and seroma. Prevention of seroma can be difficult and some surgeons leave the drains in for up to 6 weeks. [1] Ultimately if drainage output is less than 30 cc in a 24 hour period we are comfortable removing the drains with minimal concern for development of seroma. If seromas do occur, however, aspiration and sometimes treatment with doxycycline is required.

Wound separation is common, especially in the body lift procedure. While separation is usually superficial and treated with local wound care, massive tissue necrosis and dehiscence can occur. This is usually due to over resection and/or poor nutrition. Wound care, surgical debridement and negative pressure wound therapy is useful in this unfortunate situation.

Dreaded complications of venous thrombosis and pulmonary embolus should be prevented at all cost. Body contouring procedures are lengthy and post operative movement is painful, making sedentary habits even more common in these patients. For these reasons we are relatively aggressive in our protocol. First and foremost, the amount of surgery is limited to under 6-7 hours. Staging of different anatomic regions will avoid a prolonged operation, which can place the patient at higher risk for thromboembolic complications. Further, sequential compressive devices are used at all times intra-operatively and post-operatively. If the legs are in the surgical field, sterile compression devices are utilized. Early ambulation is a requirement for all of our patients. Finally, low molecular weight heparin is started post operative day one after evaluation by the surgeon. This is generally continued for 7 days after any significant body contouring procedure except for those involving the facial region.

References

[1] Aly, A. S. (2006) Belt Lipectomy. In Aly, A. S. *Body Contouring After Massive Weight Loss*. (pp 72-145). St. Louis, MO: Quality Medical Publishing, Inc.

[2] Aly, A. S., Cram A. E. (2006) Brachioplasty. In Aly, A. S. *Body Contouring After Massive Weight Loss*. (pp 304-333). St. Louis, MO: Quality Medical Publishing, Inc.

Index

A

B

C

D

E

F

G

H

I

N

O

P

T

U

V

W

Y

Z